This Book Belongs To:

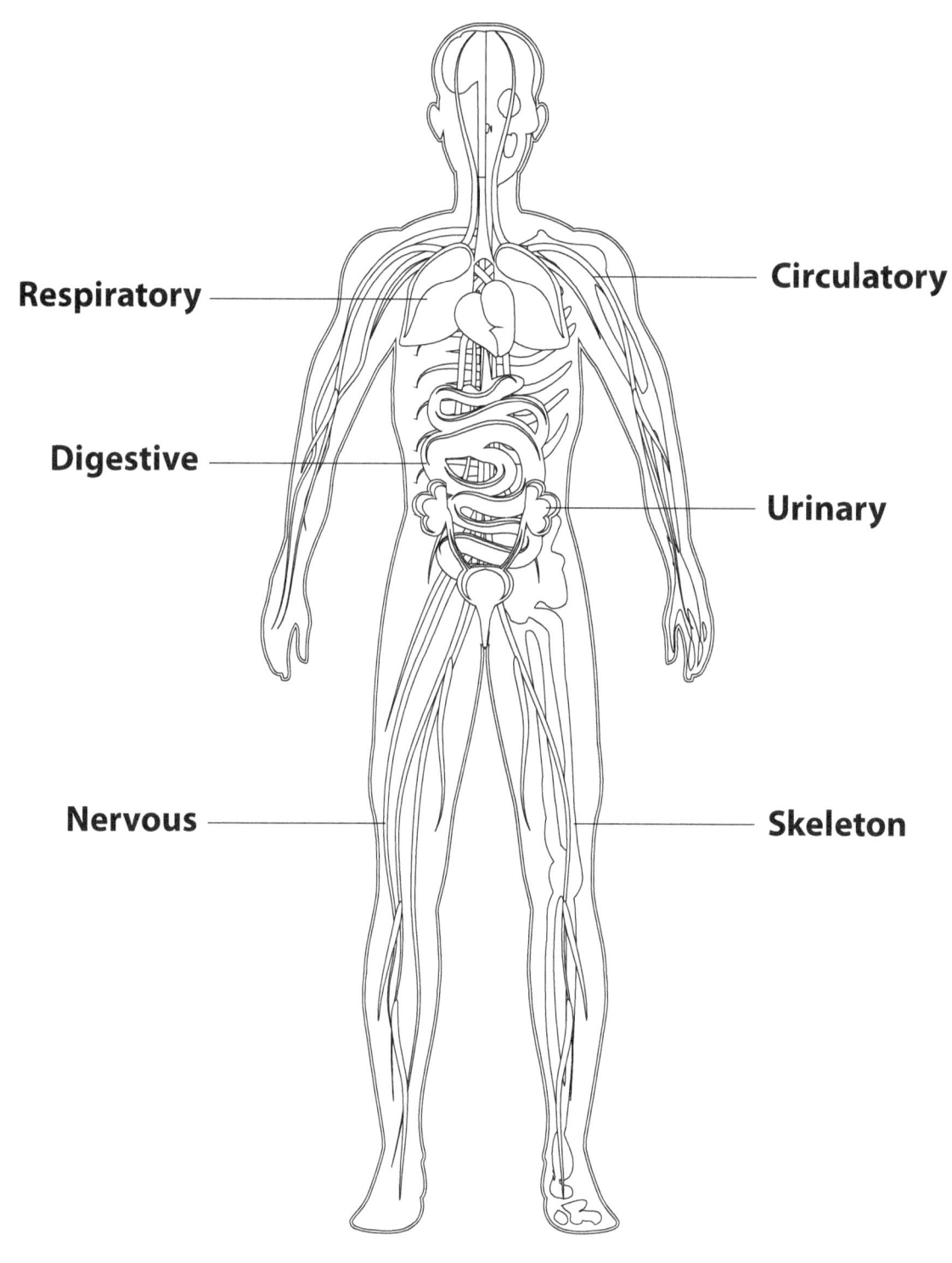

Respiratory

Circulatory

Digestive

Urinary

Nervous

Skeleton

Human Anatomy

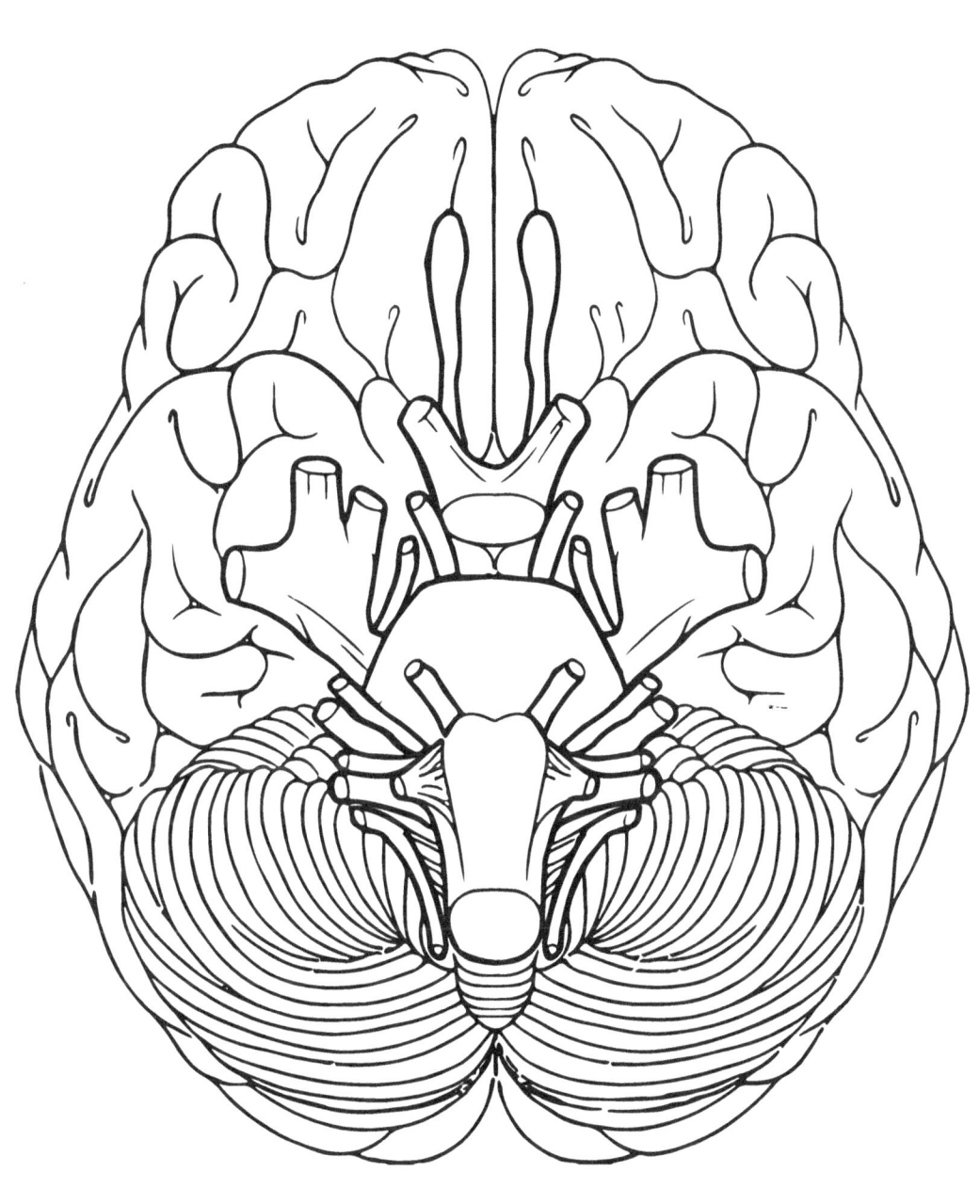

Brain

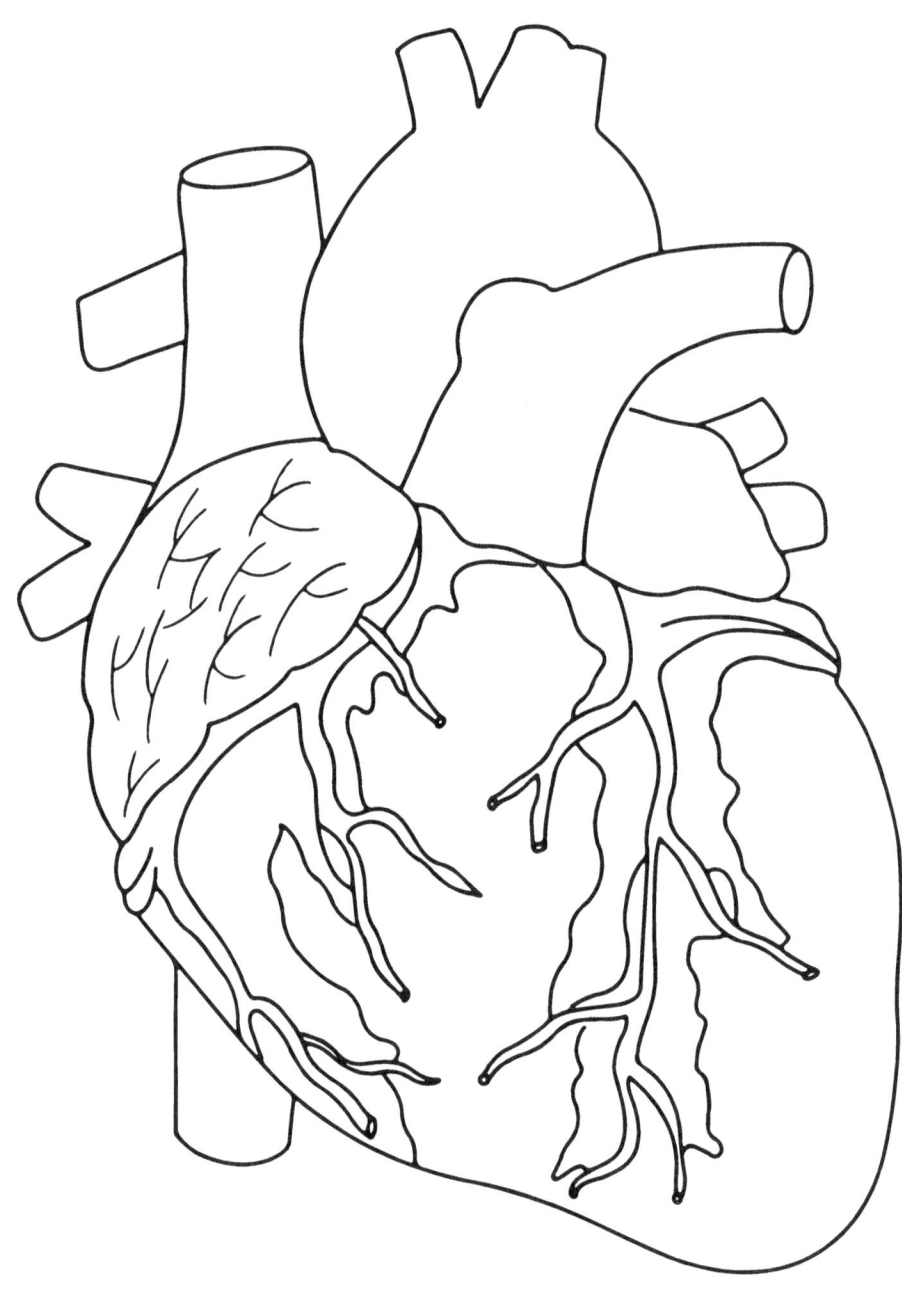

Heart

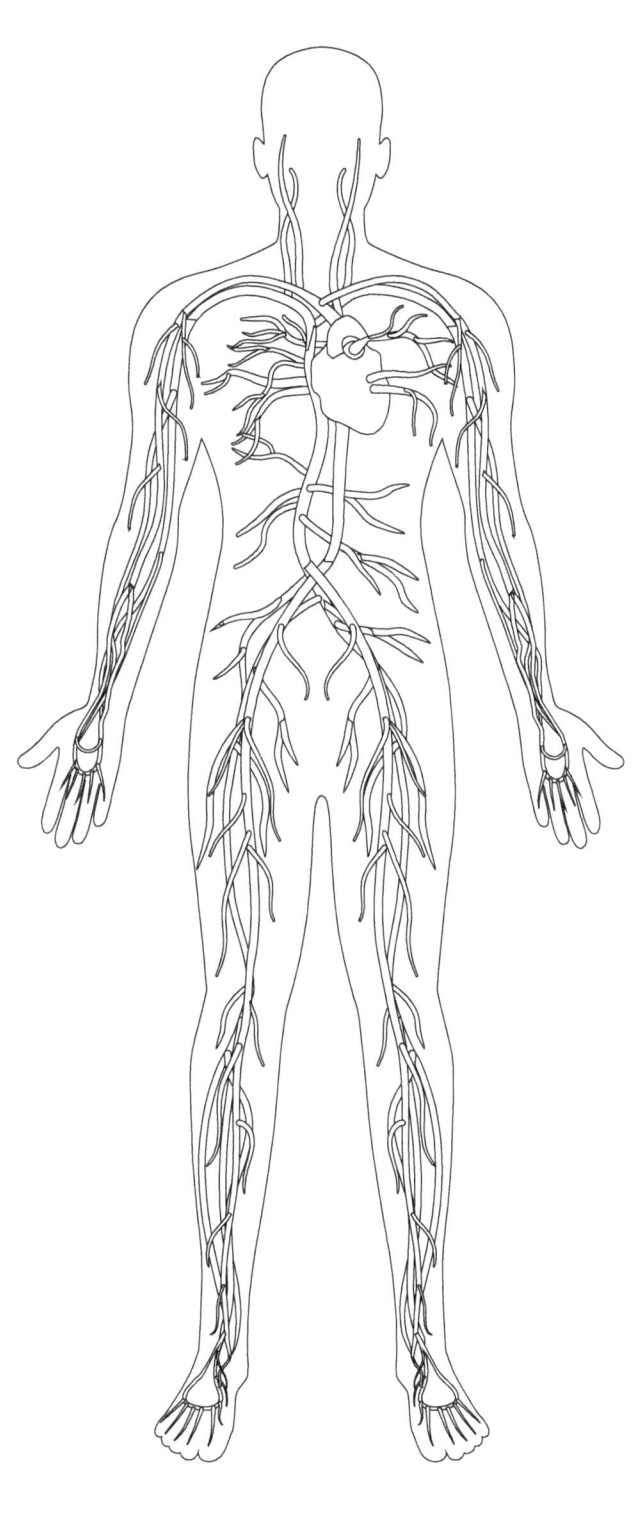

Circulatory System

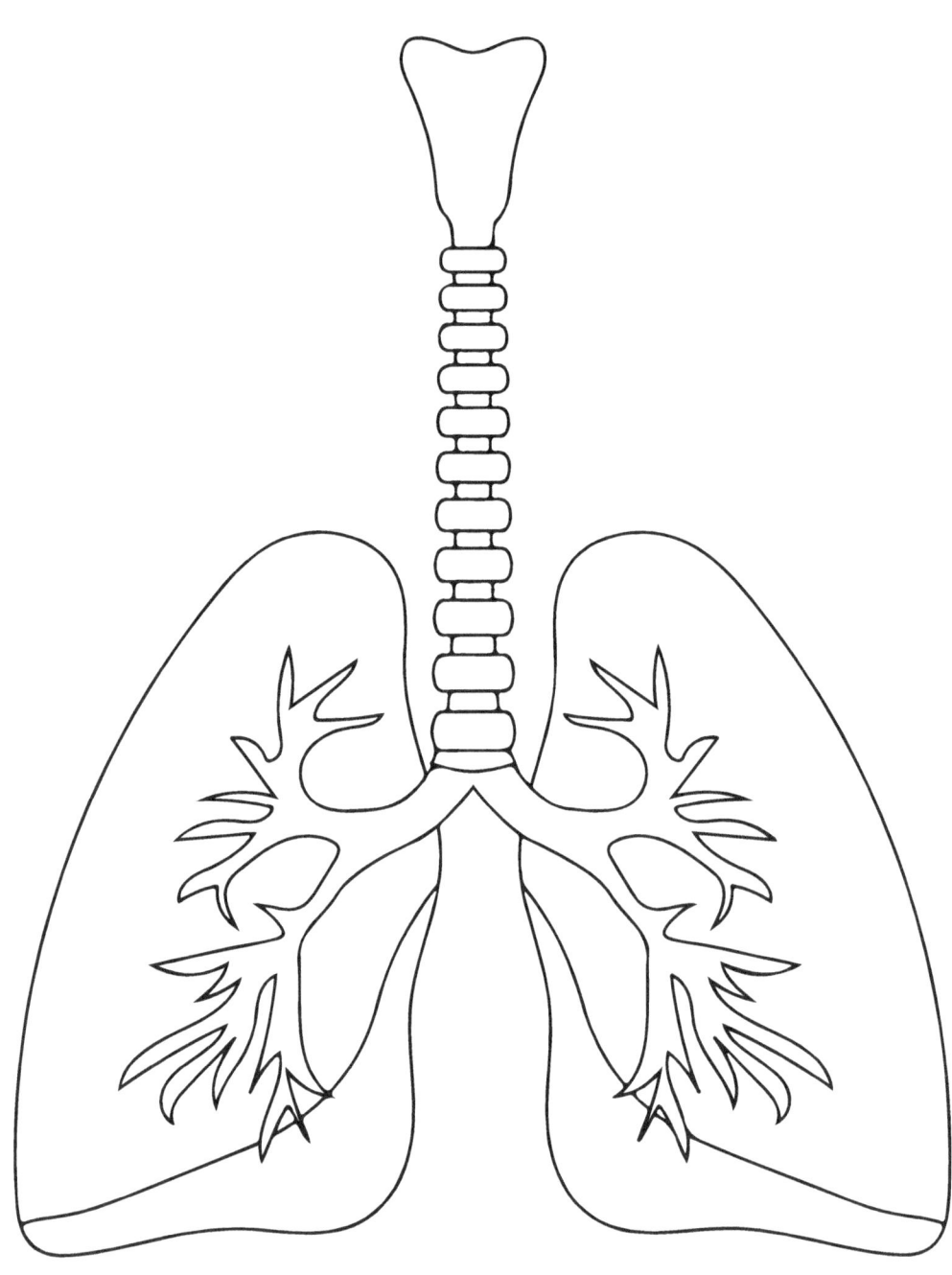

Lungs

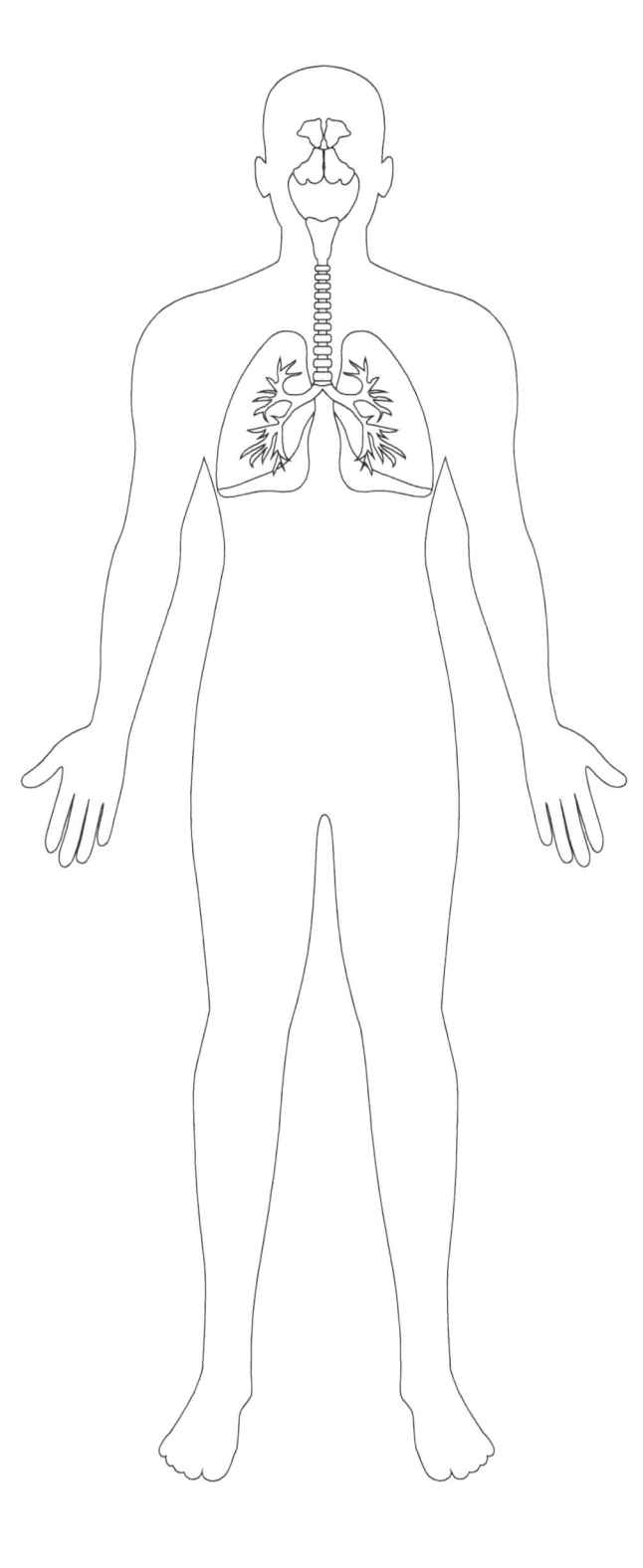

Respiratory System

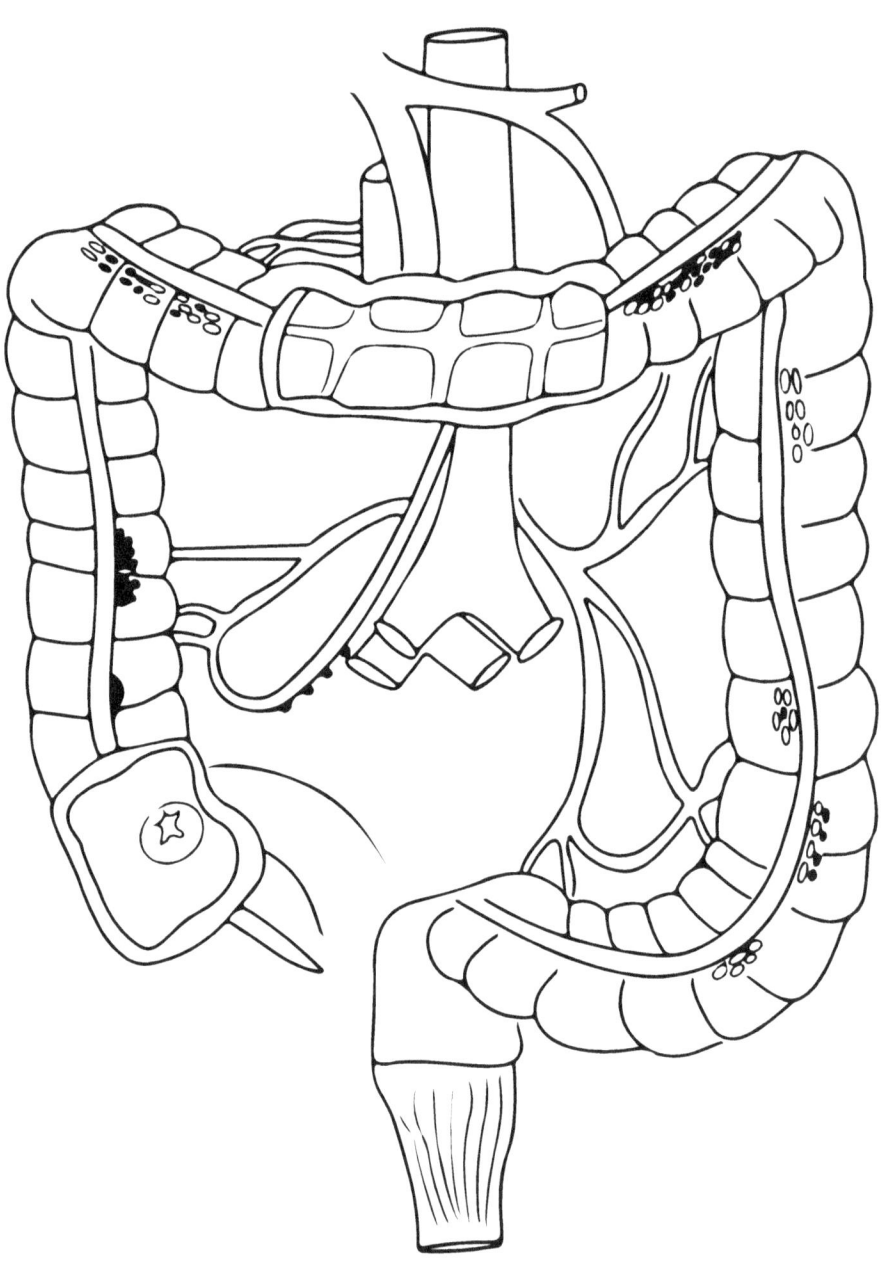

Intestine

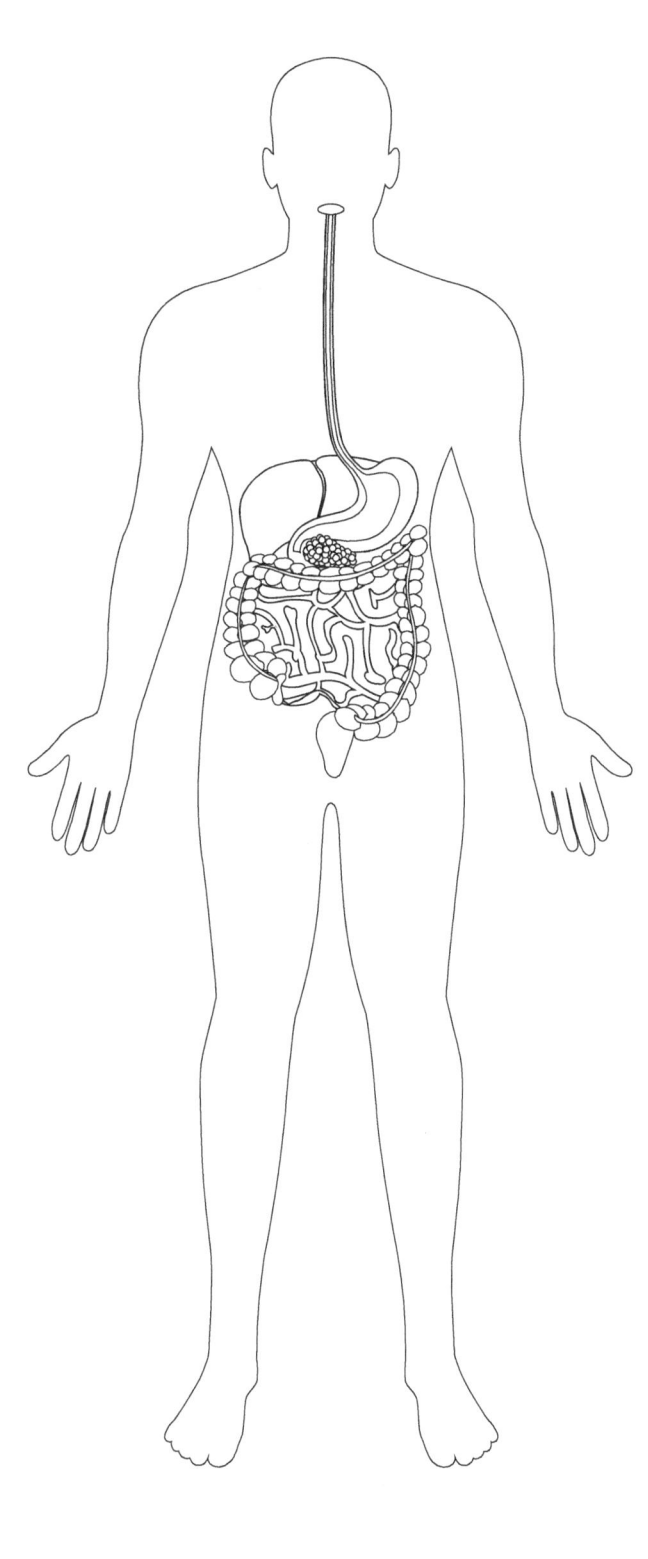

Digestive System

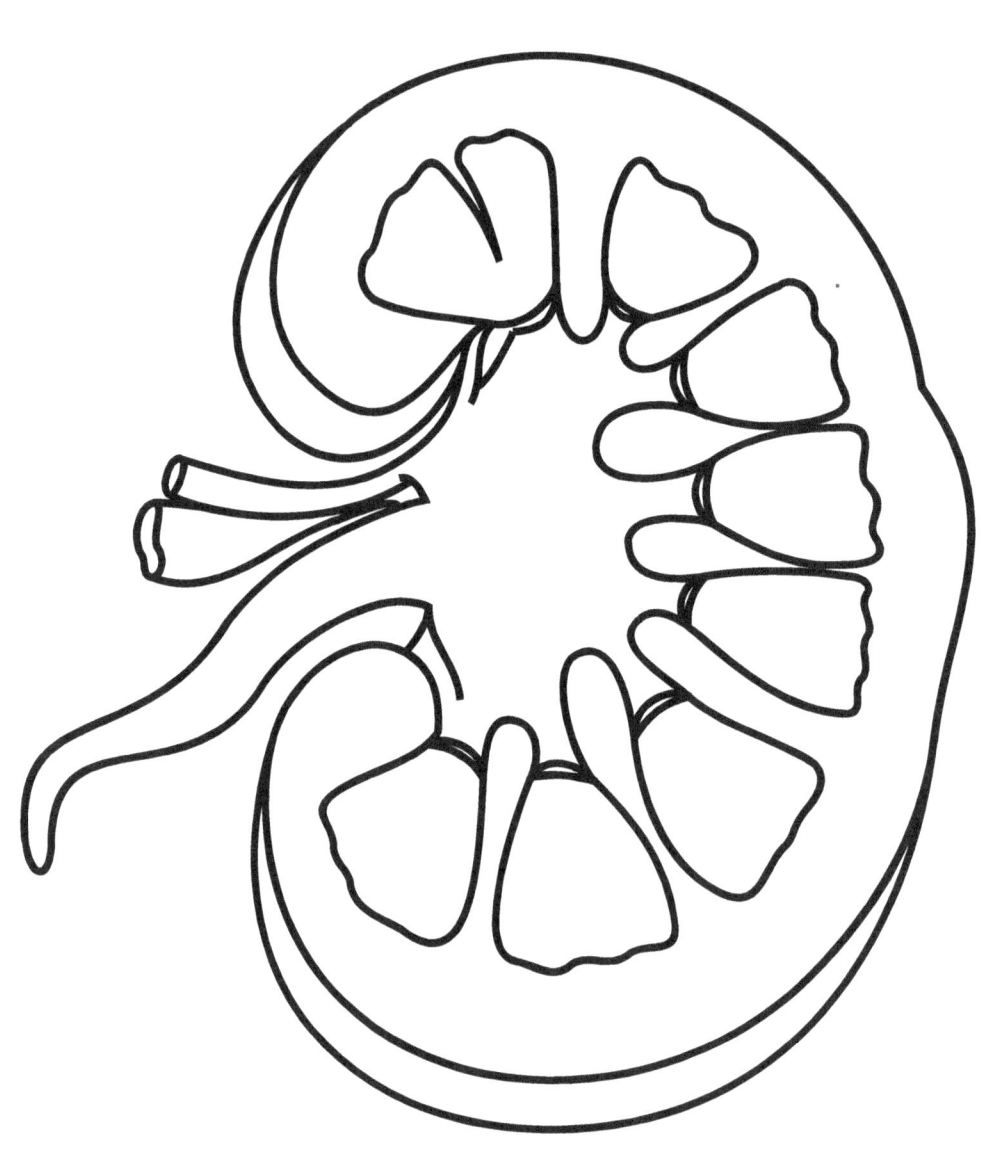

Kidney

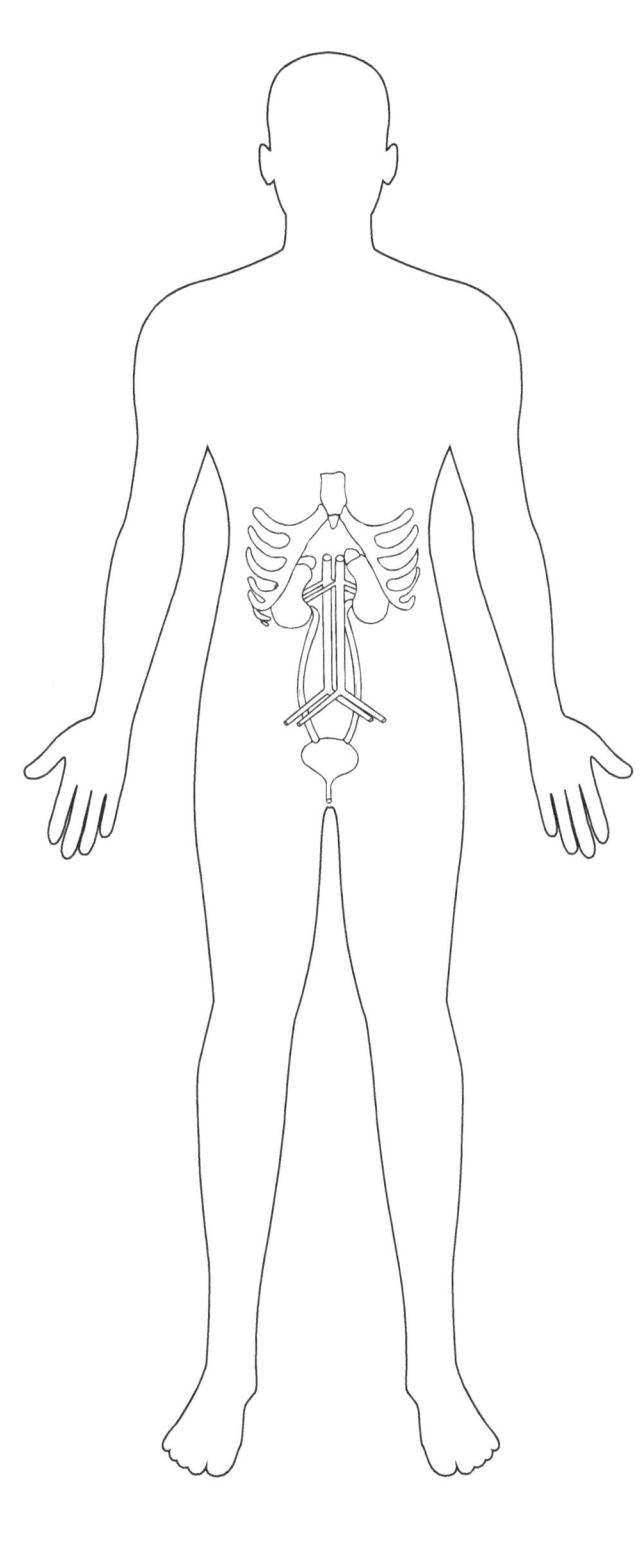

Urinary System

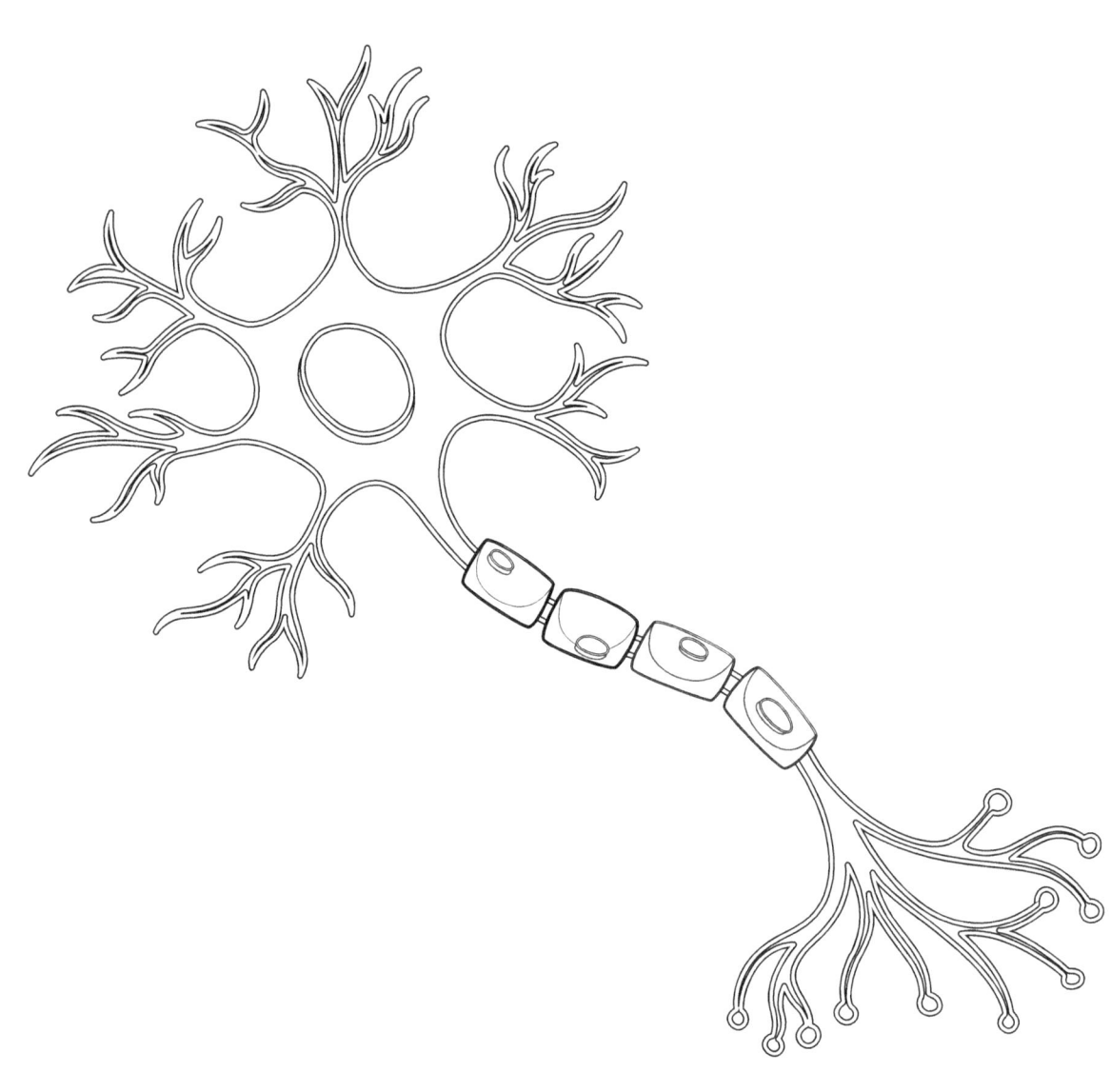

Nerve Cell

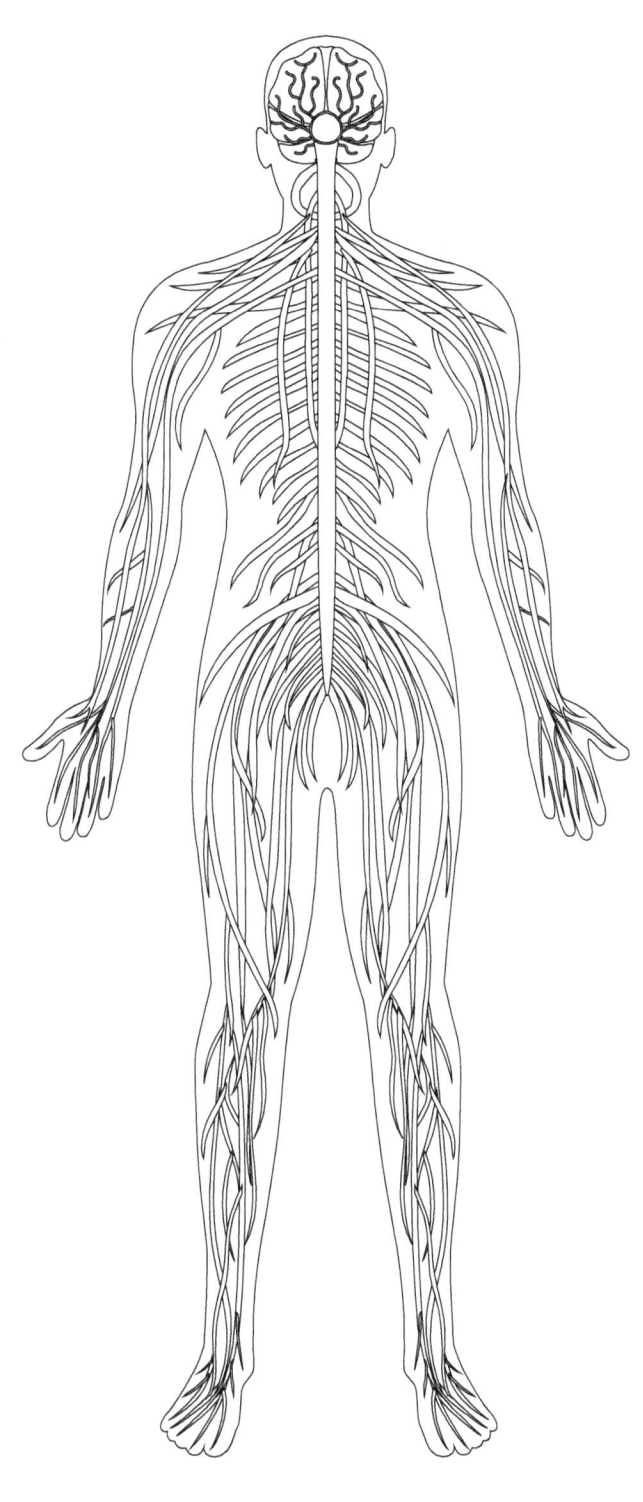

Nervous System

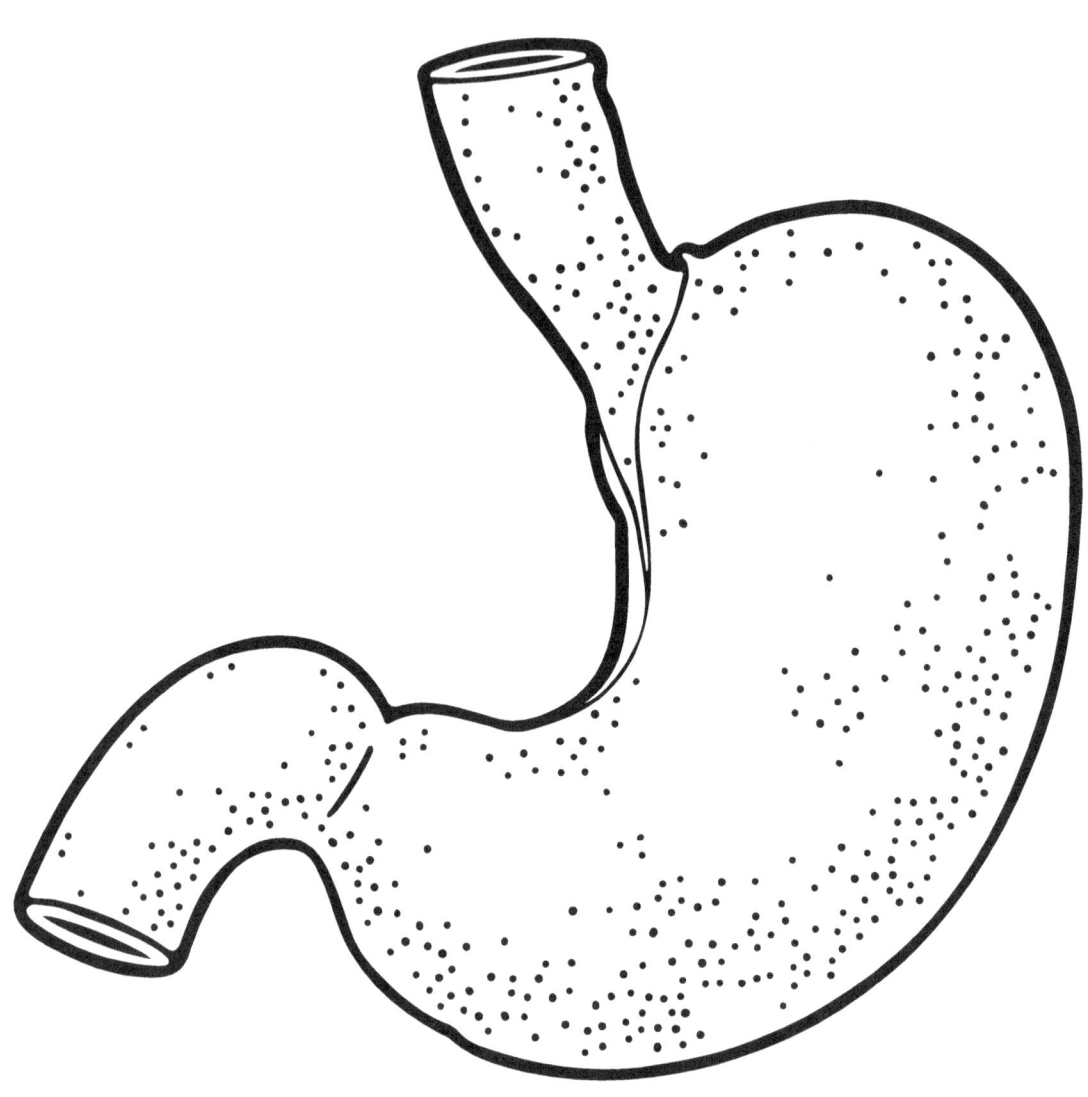

Stomach

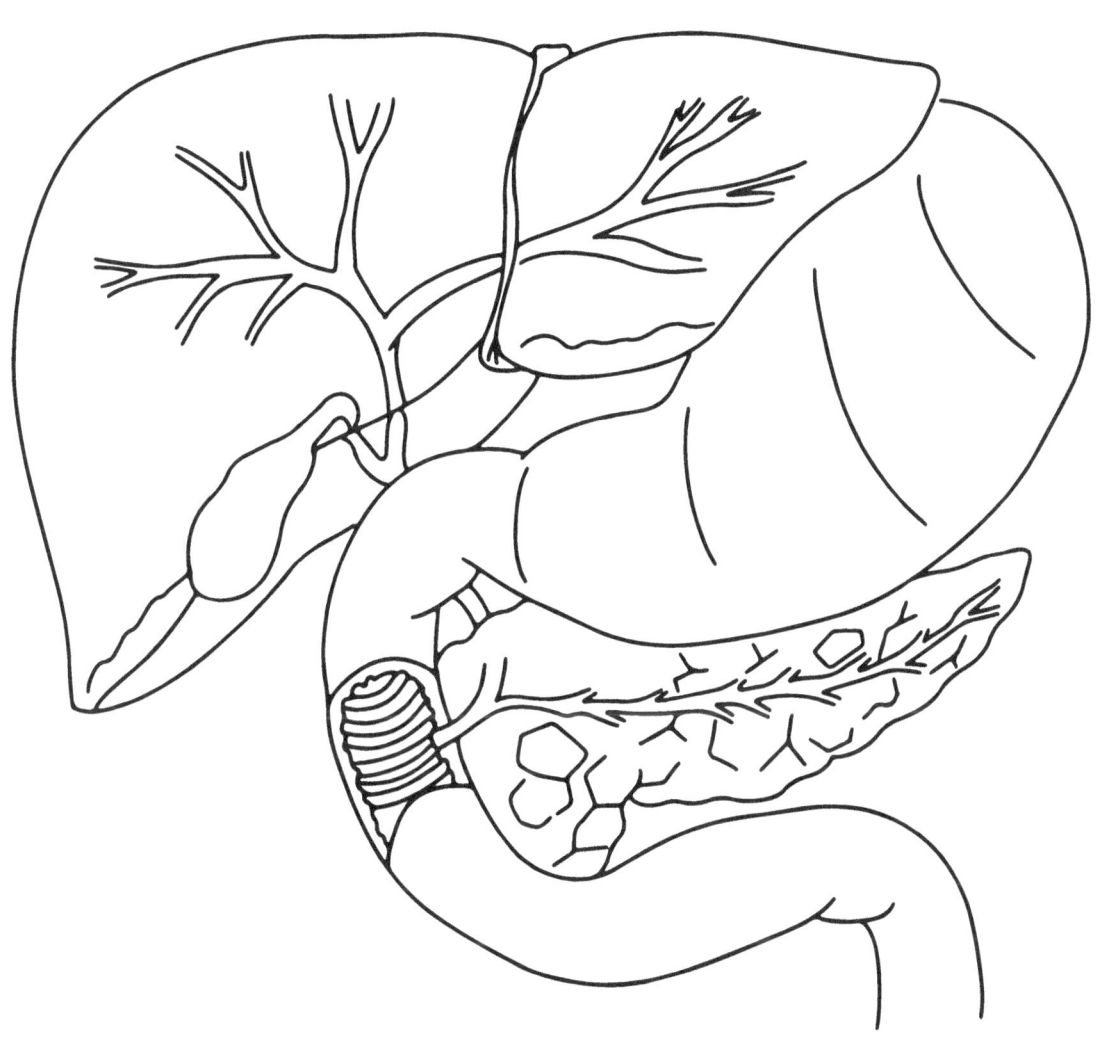

Liver

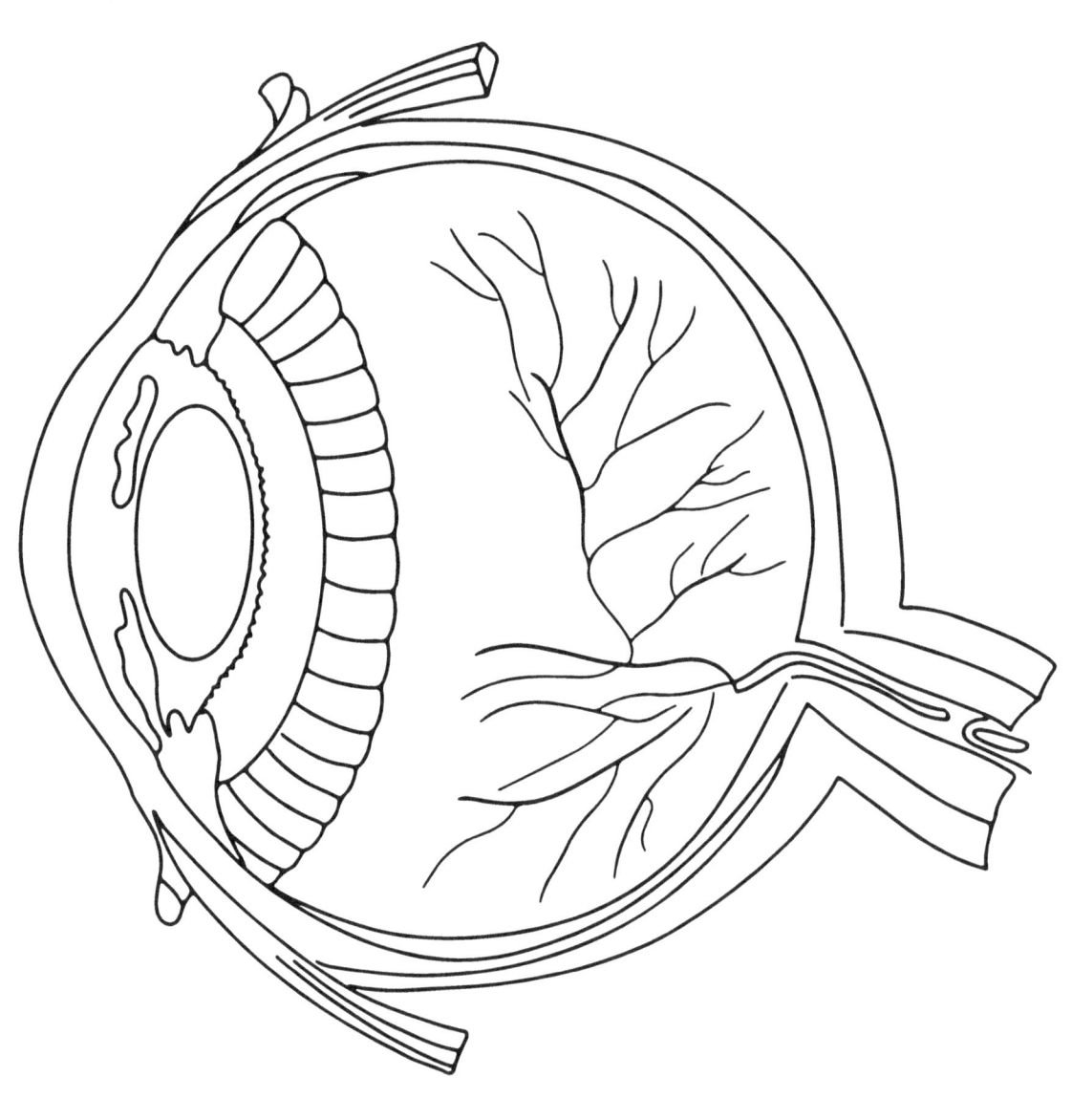

Eye

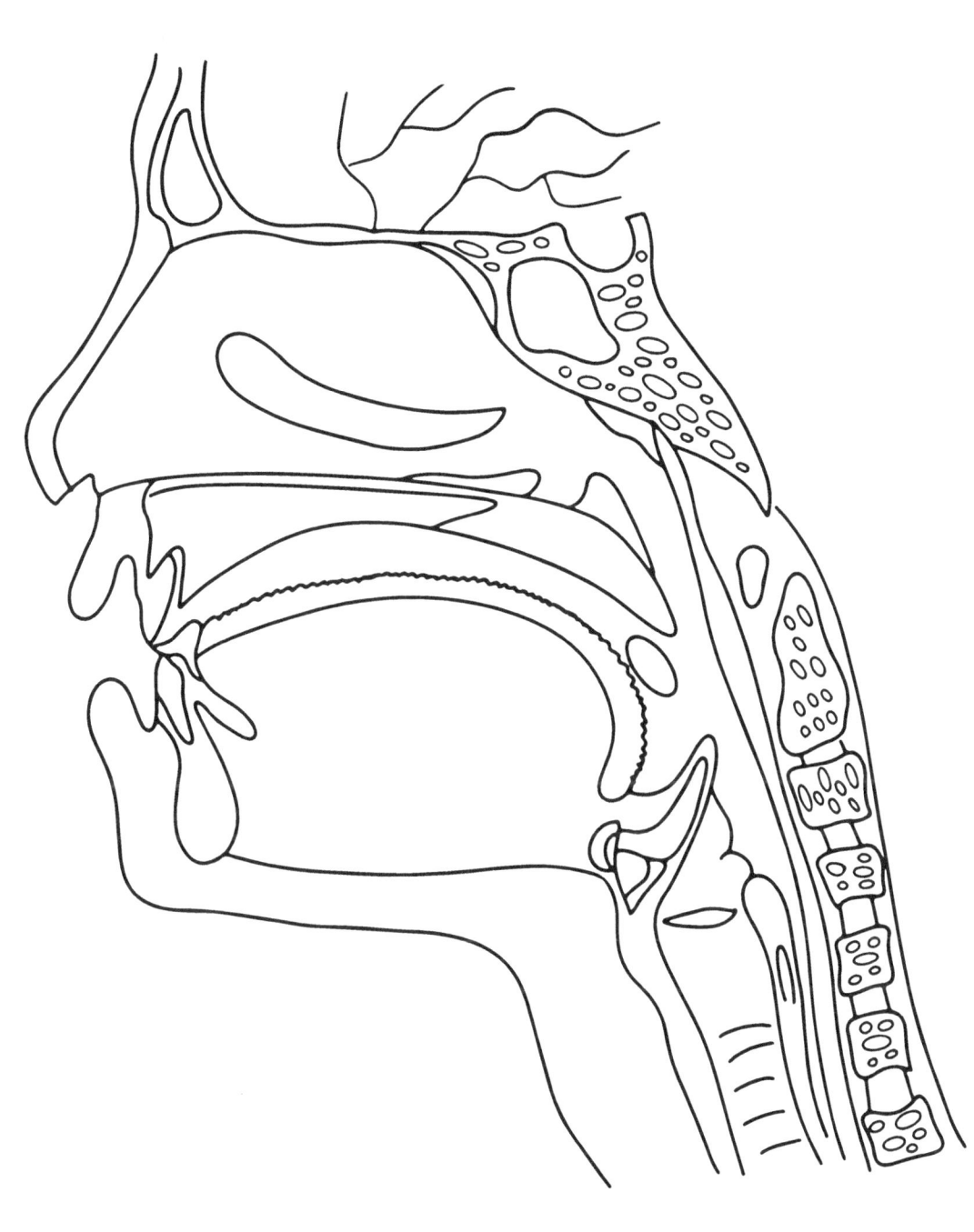

Nose and Throat

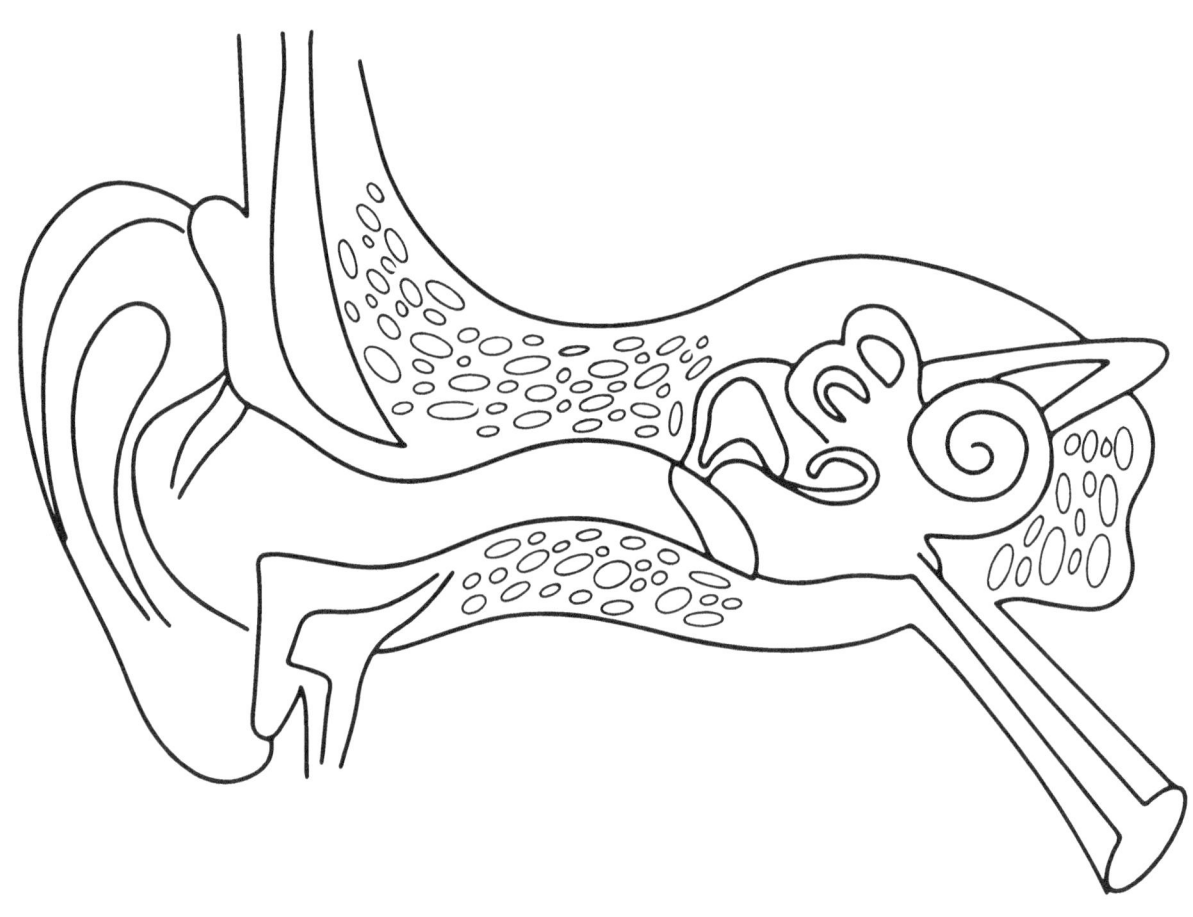

Ear

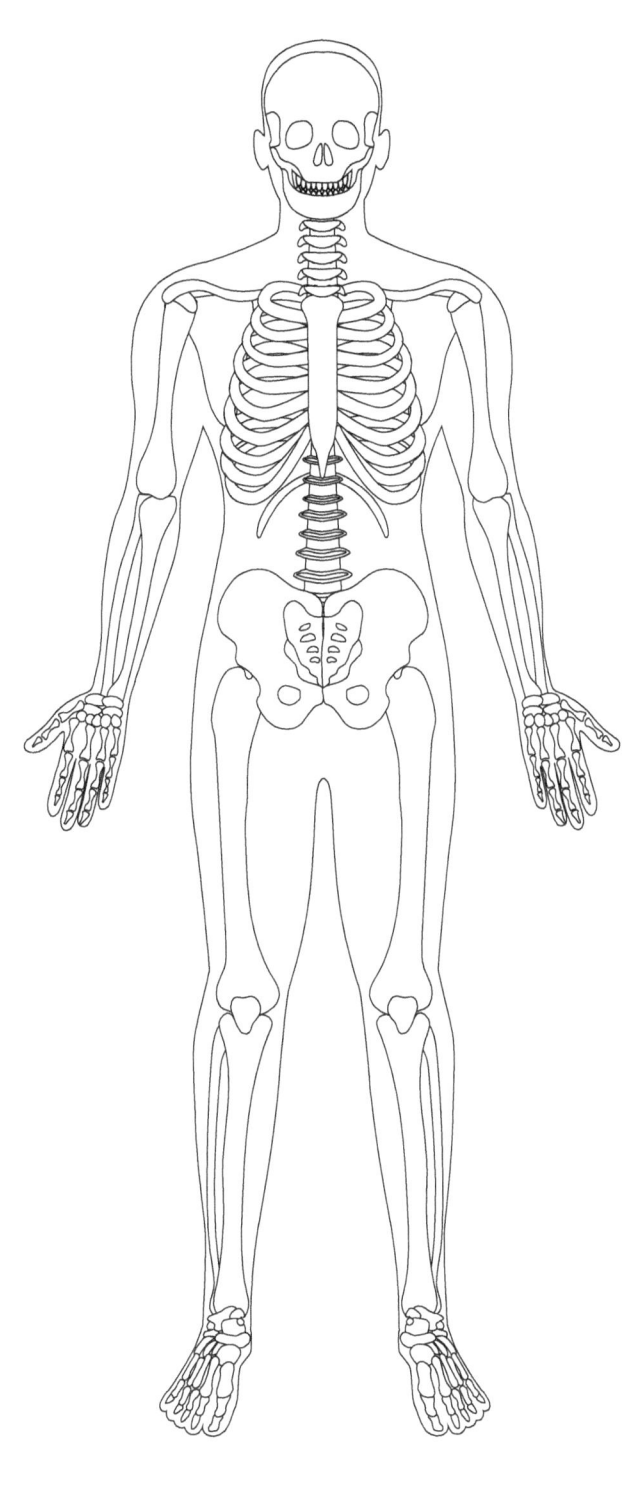

Skeletal System

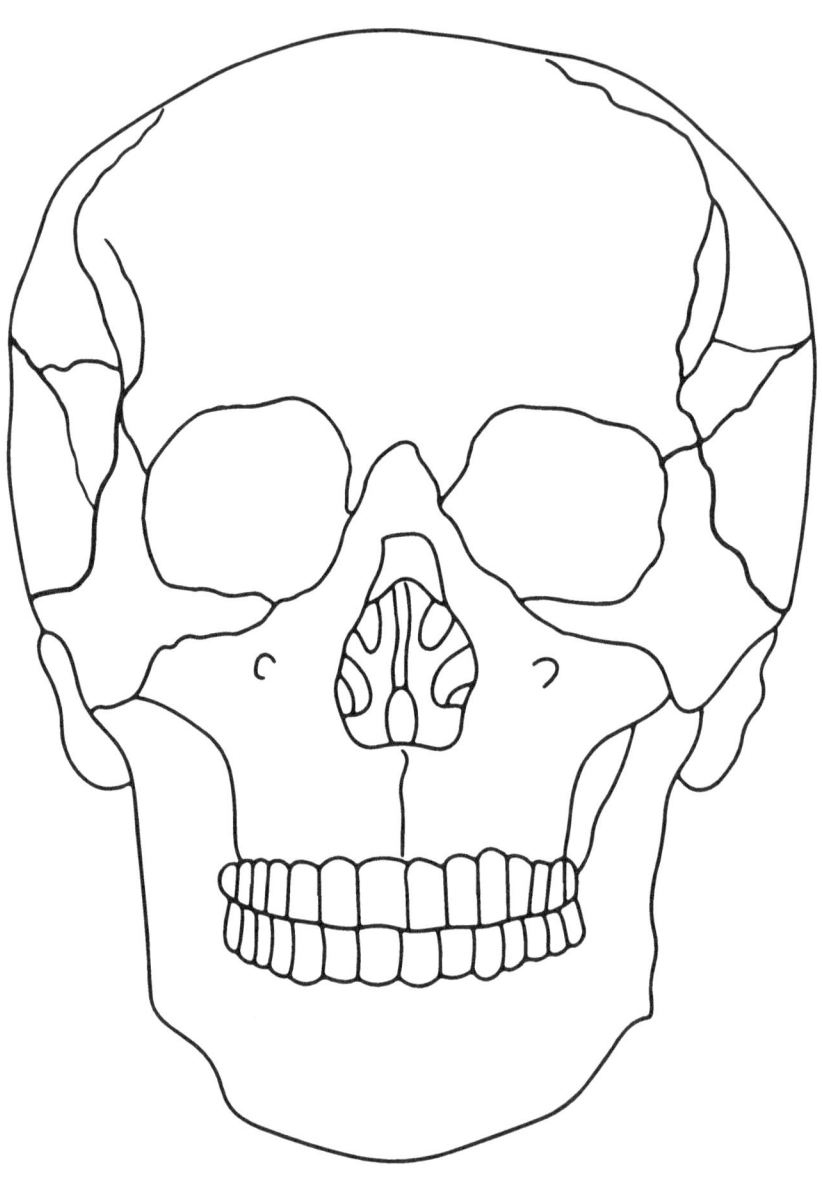

Skull

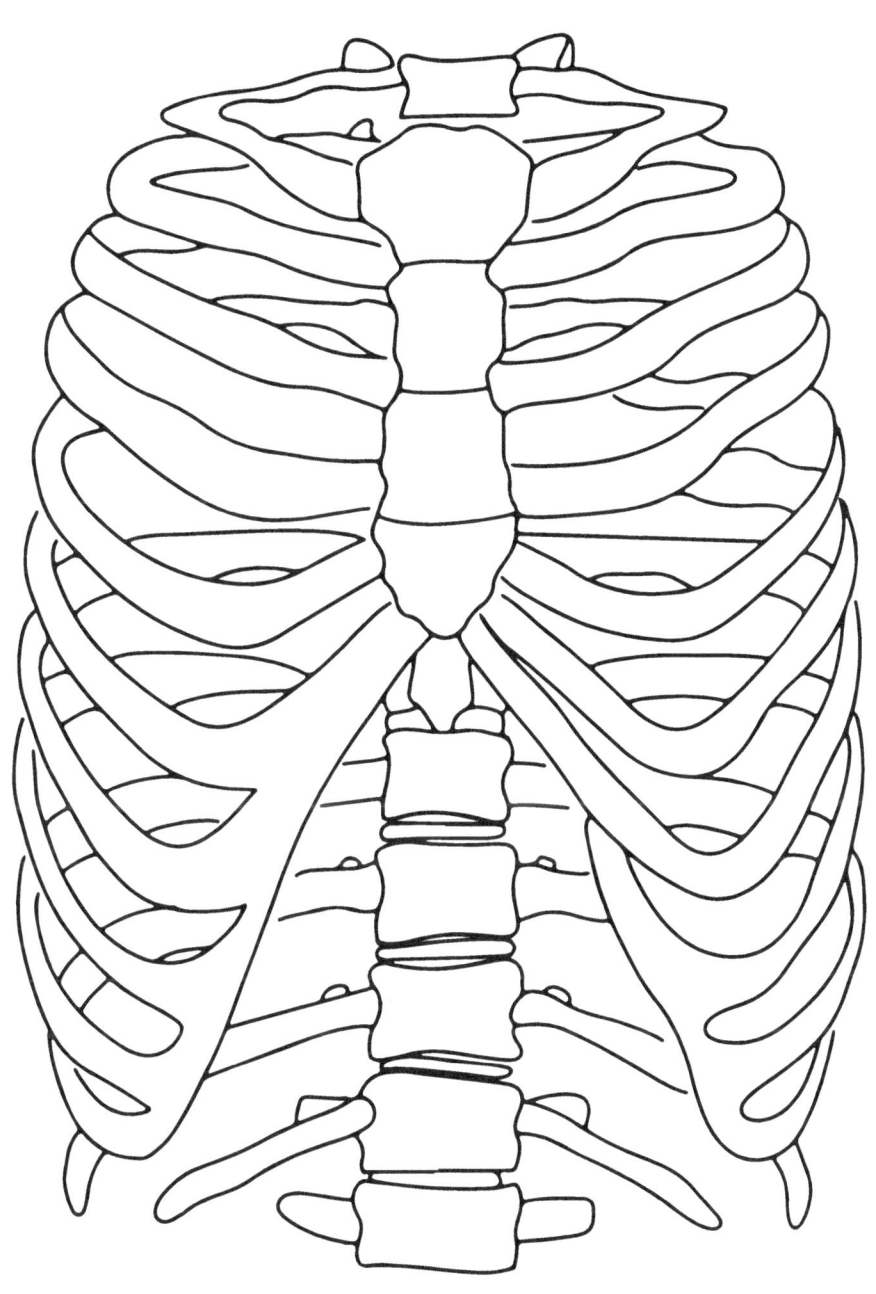

Ribs

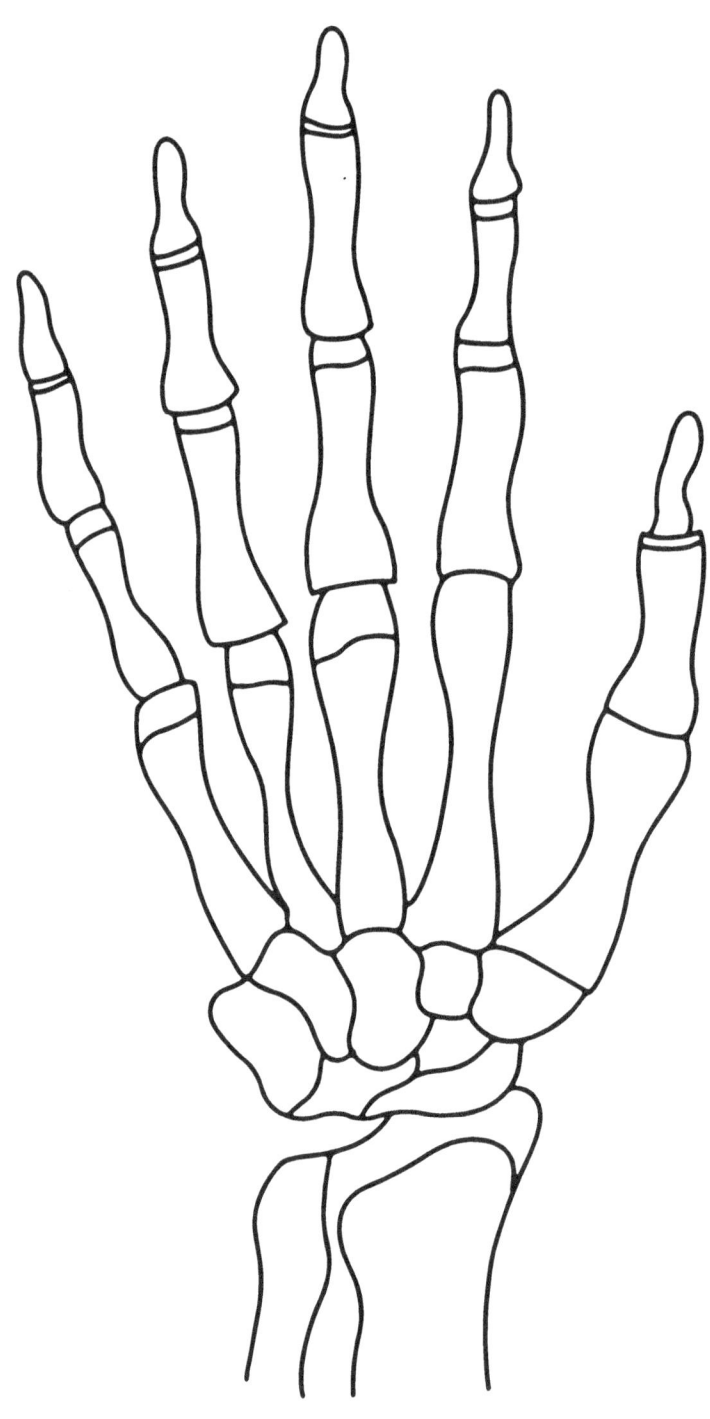

Hand and Wrist

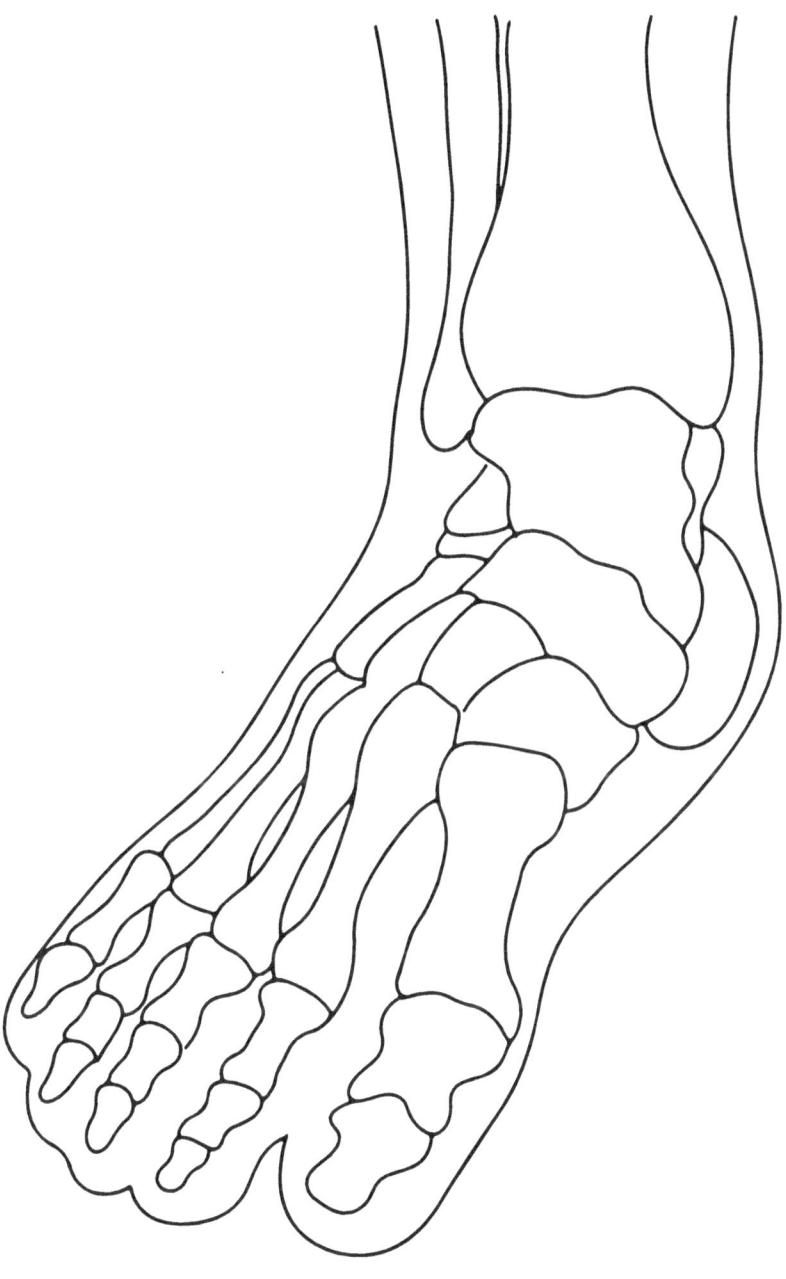

Leg

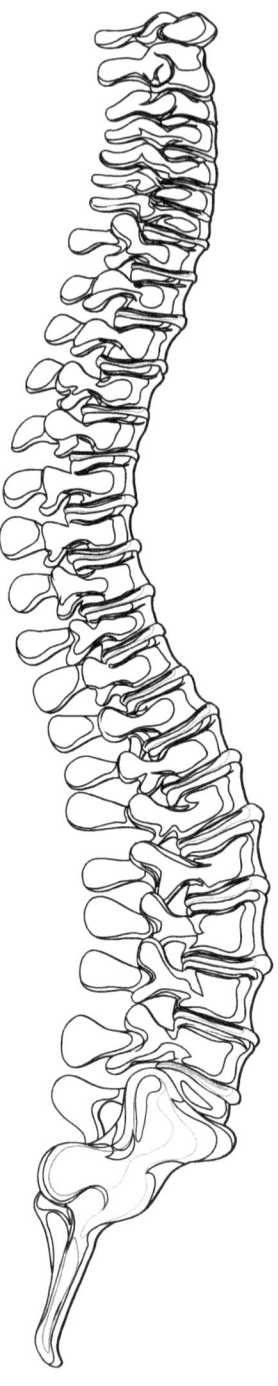

Spine

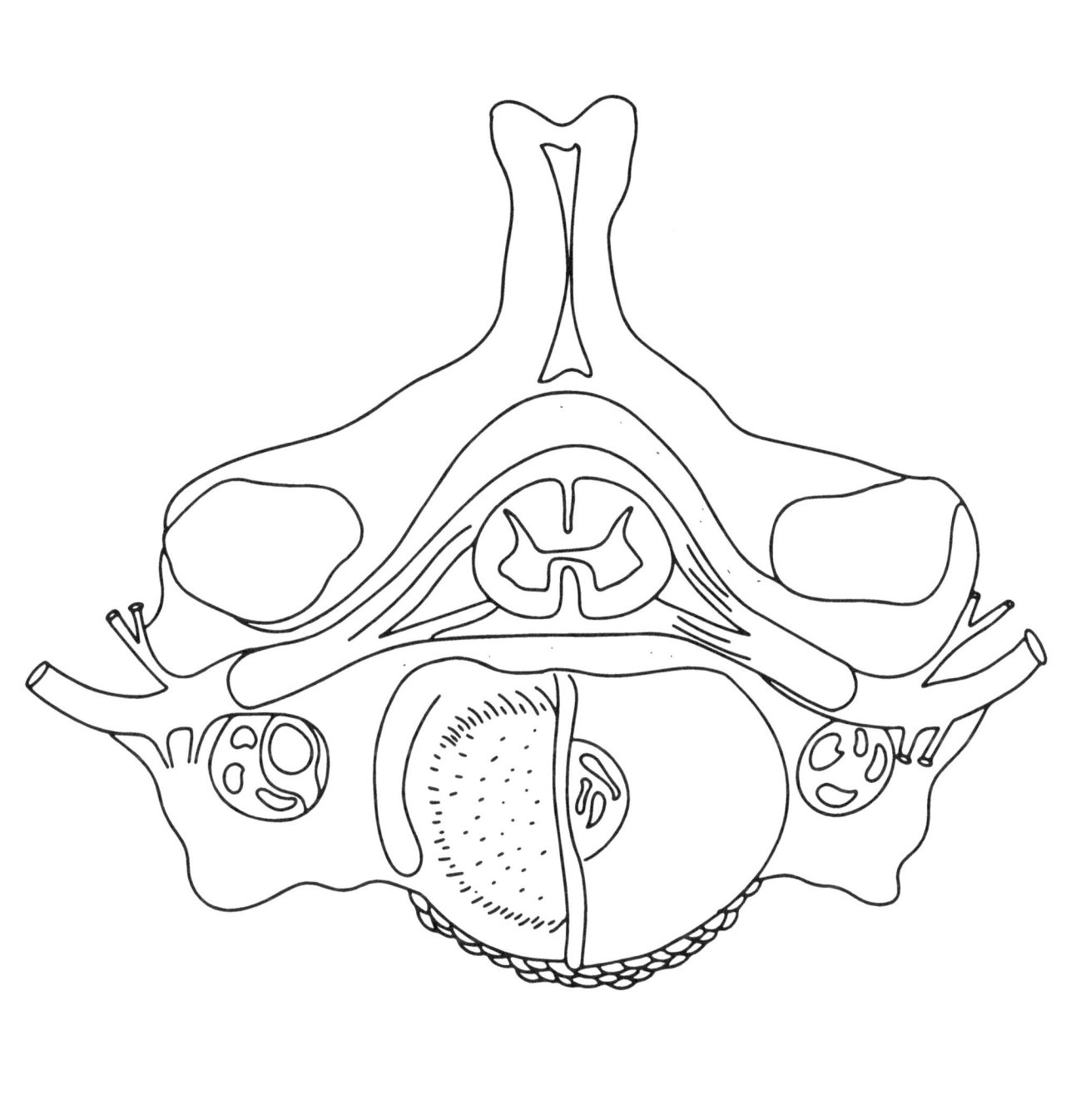

Spinal Cord

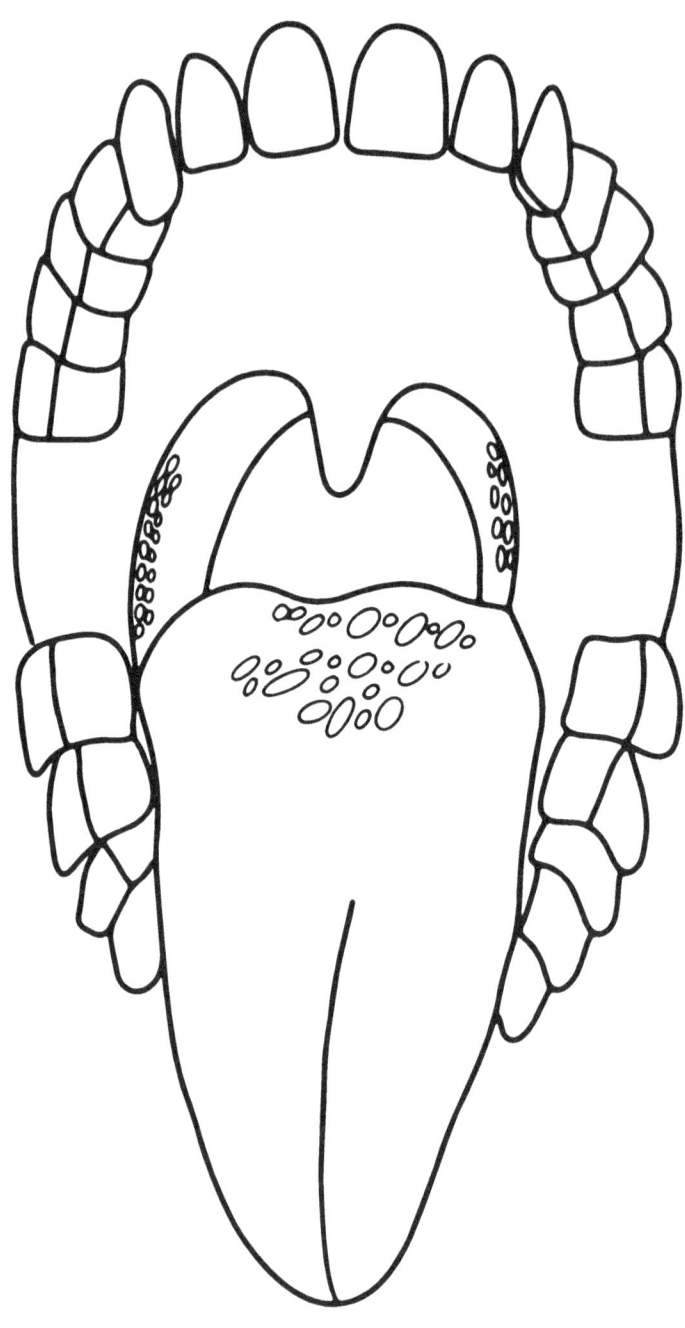

Tongue

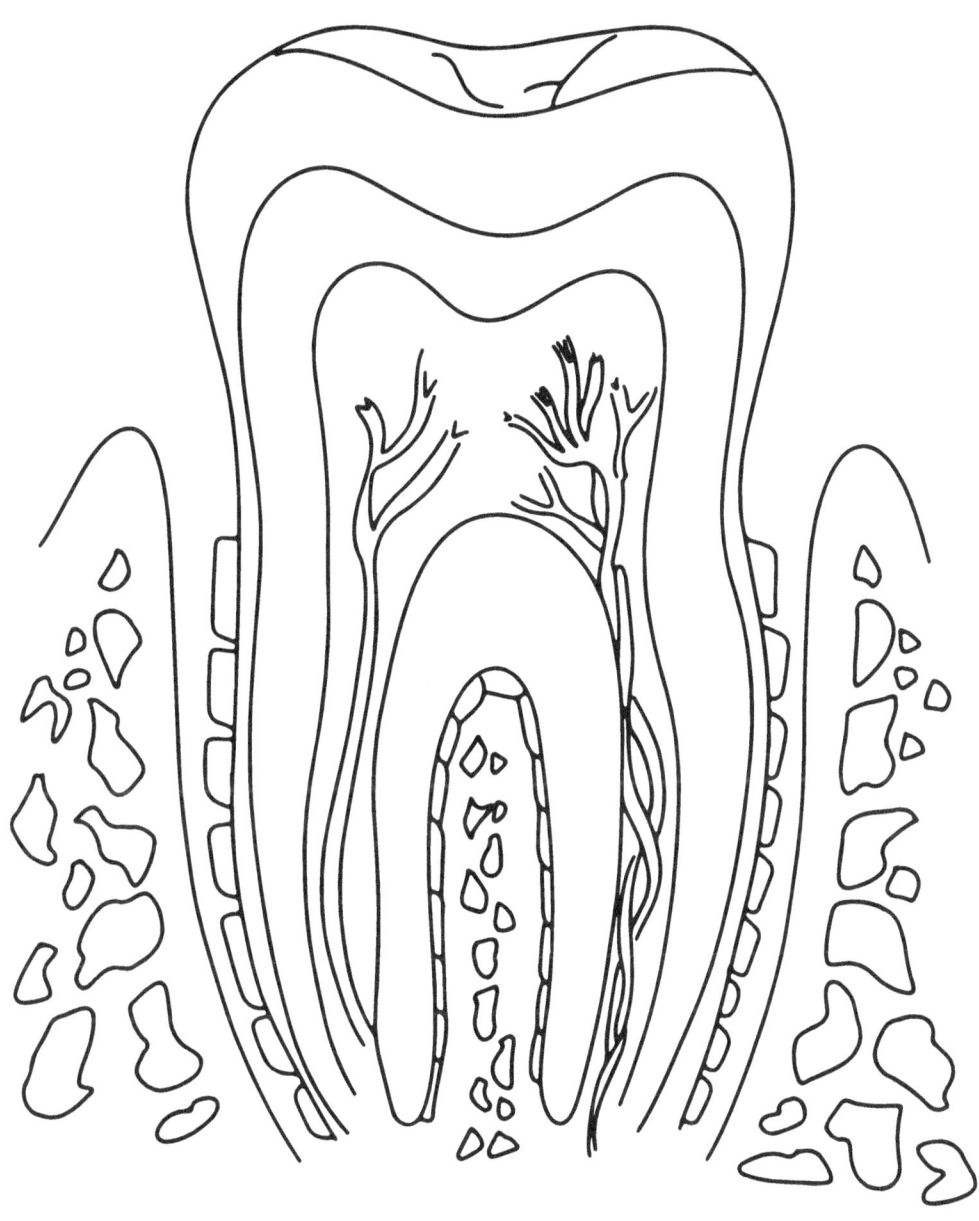

Teeth Structure

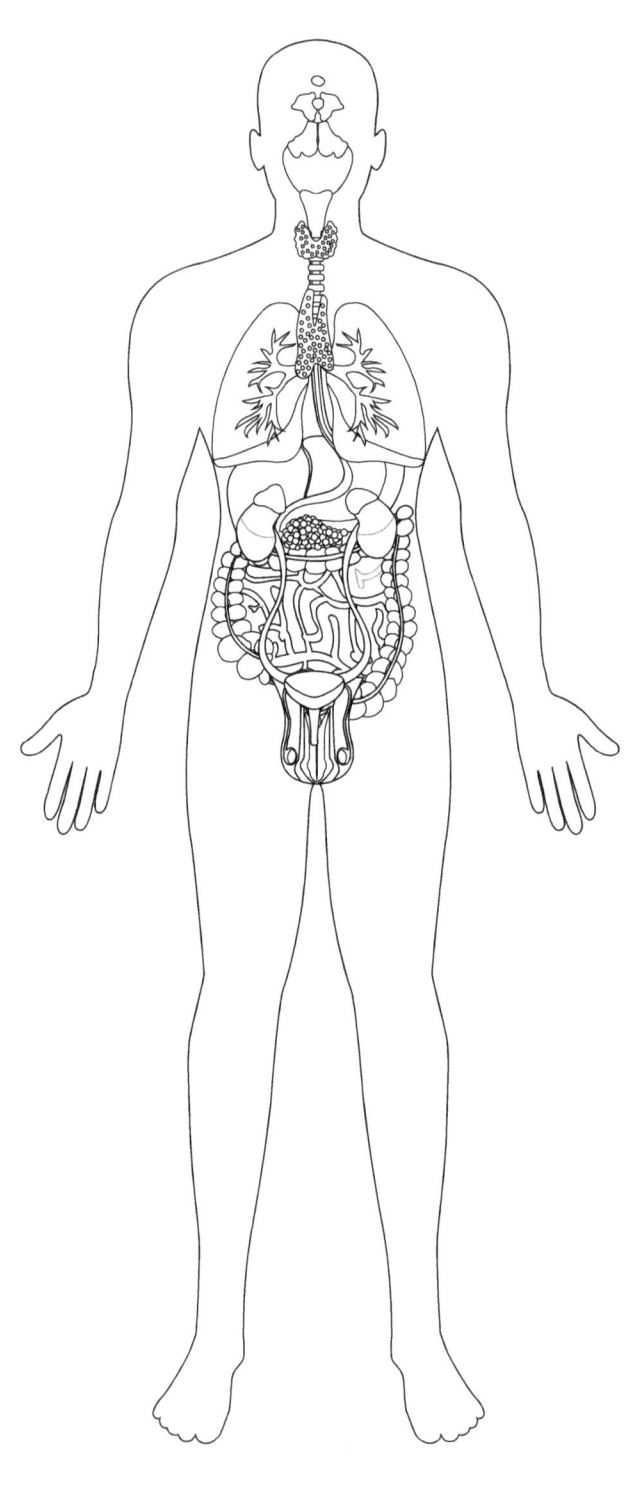

Internal Oragns

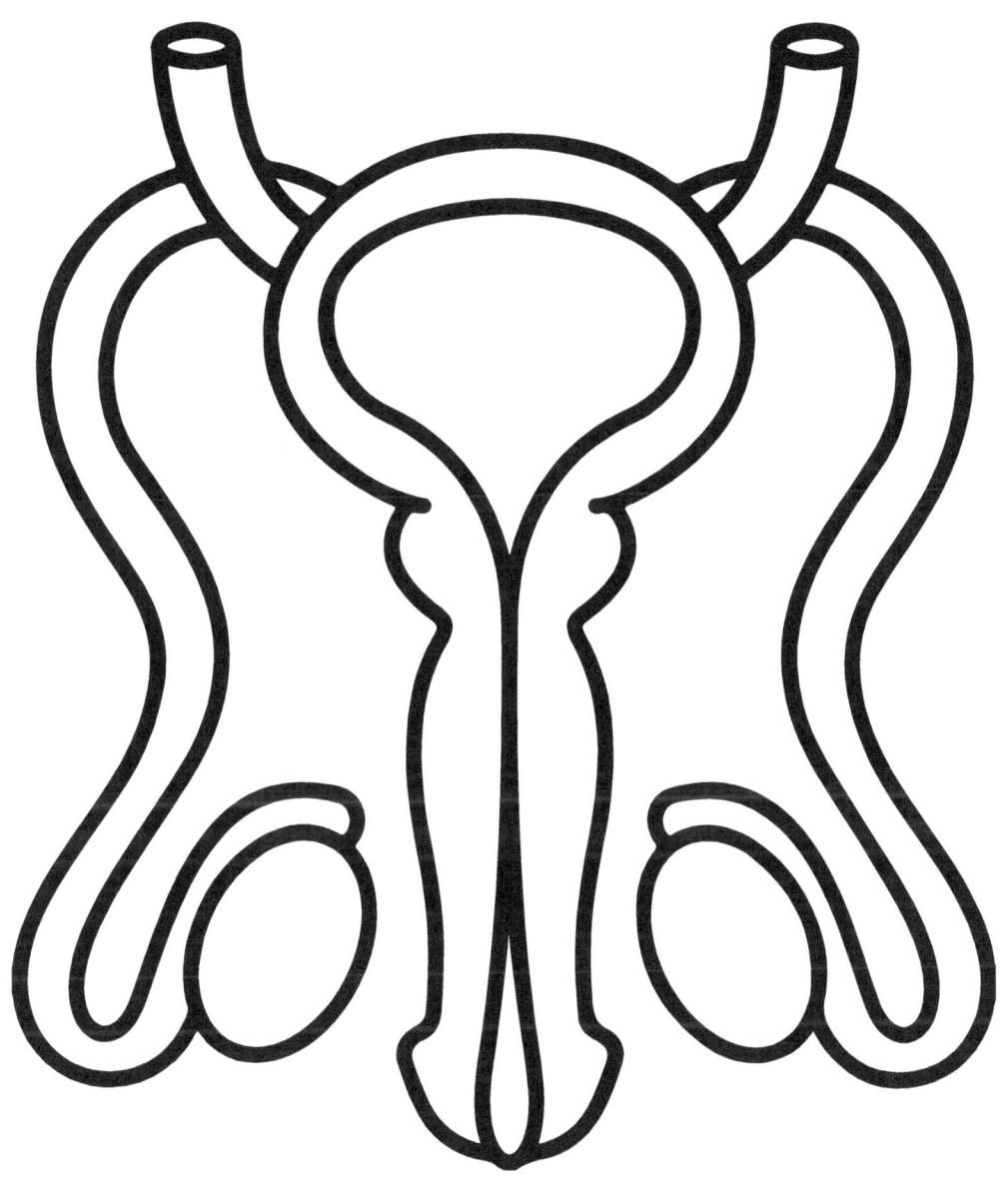

Male Reproductive System

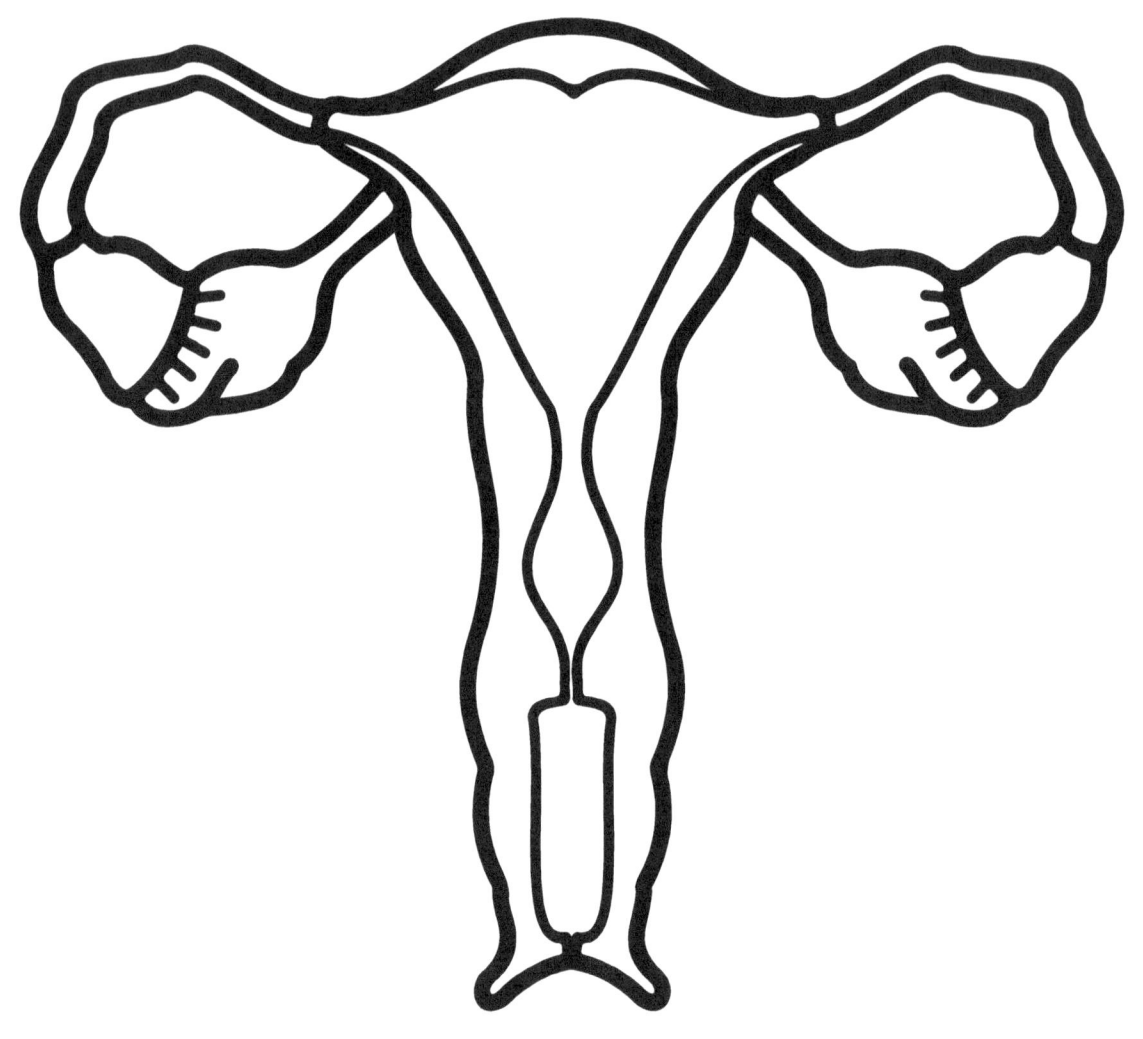

Female Reproductive System

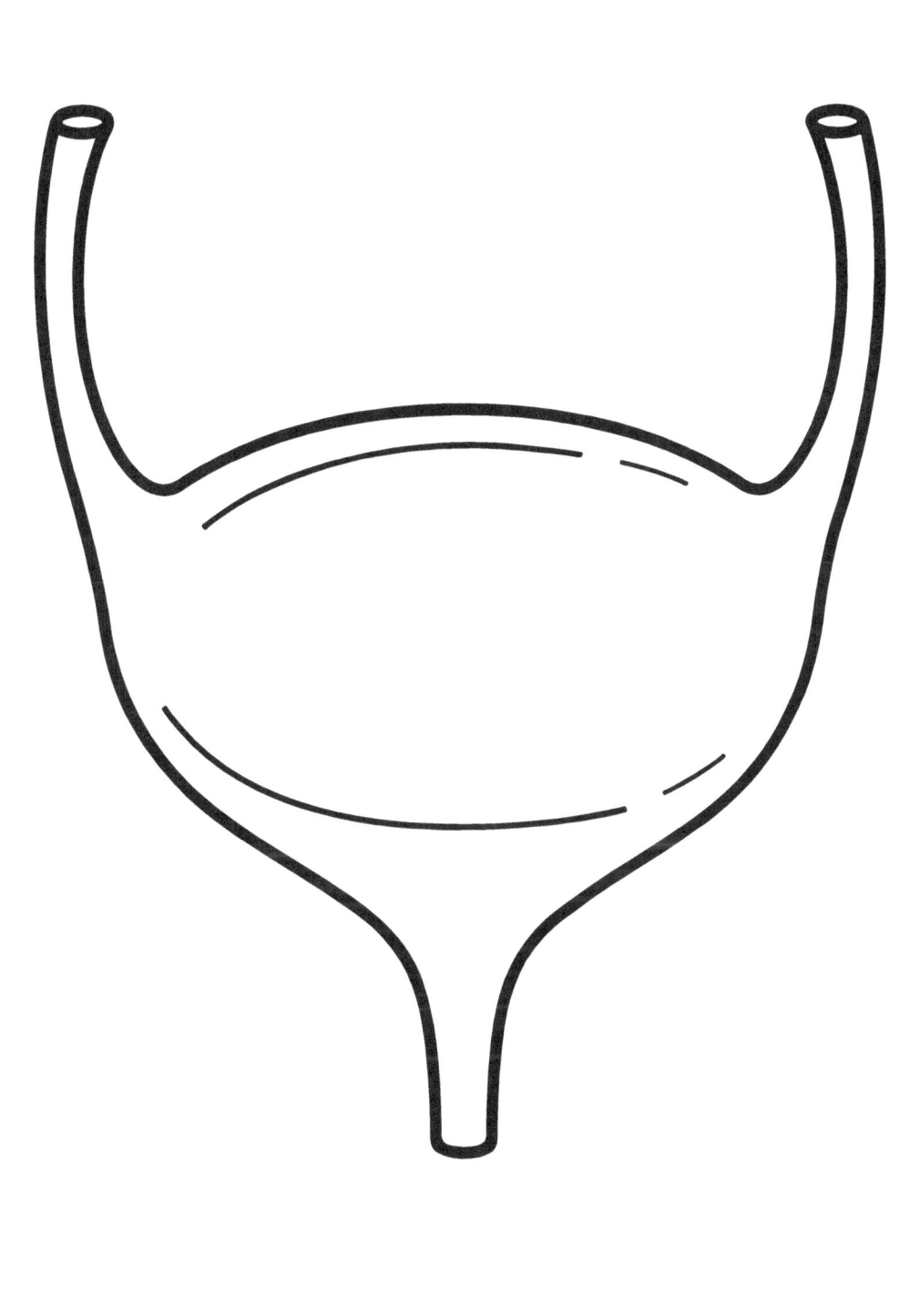

Bladder

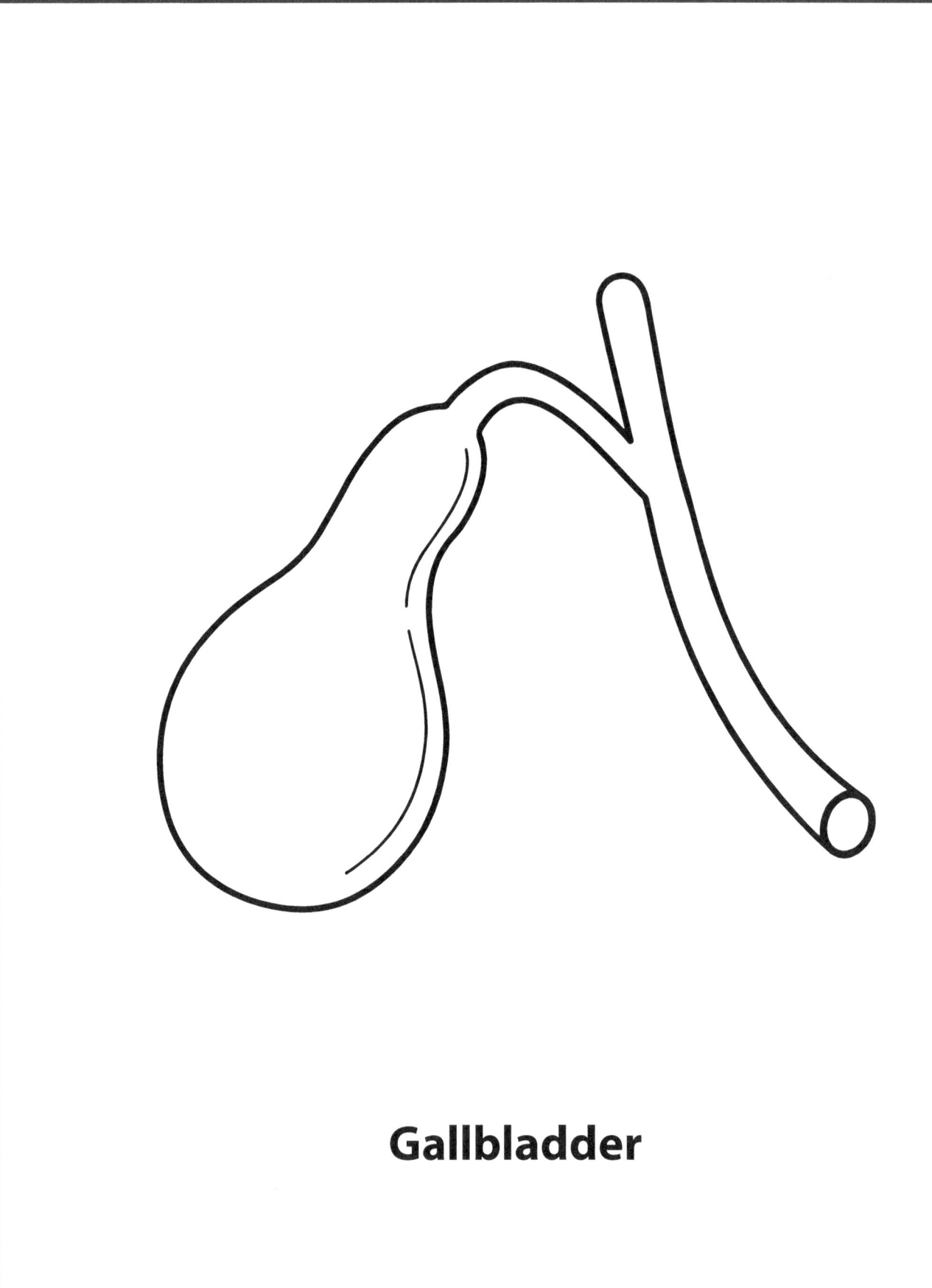

Gallbladder

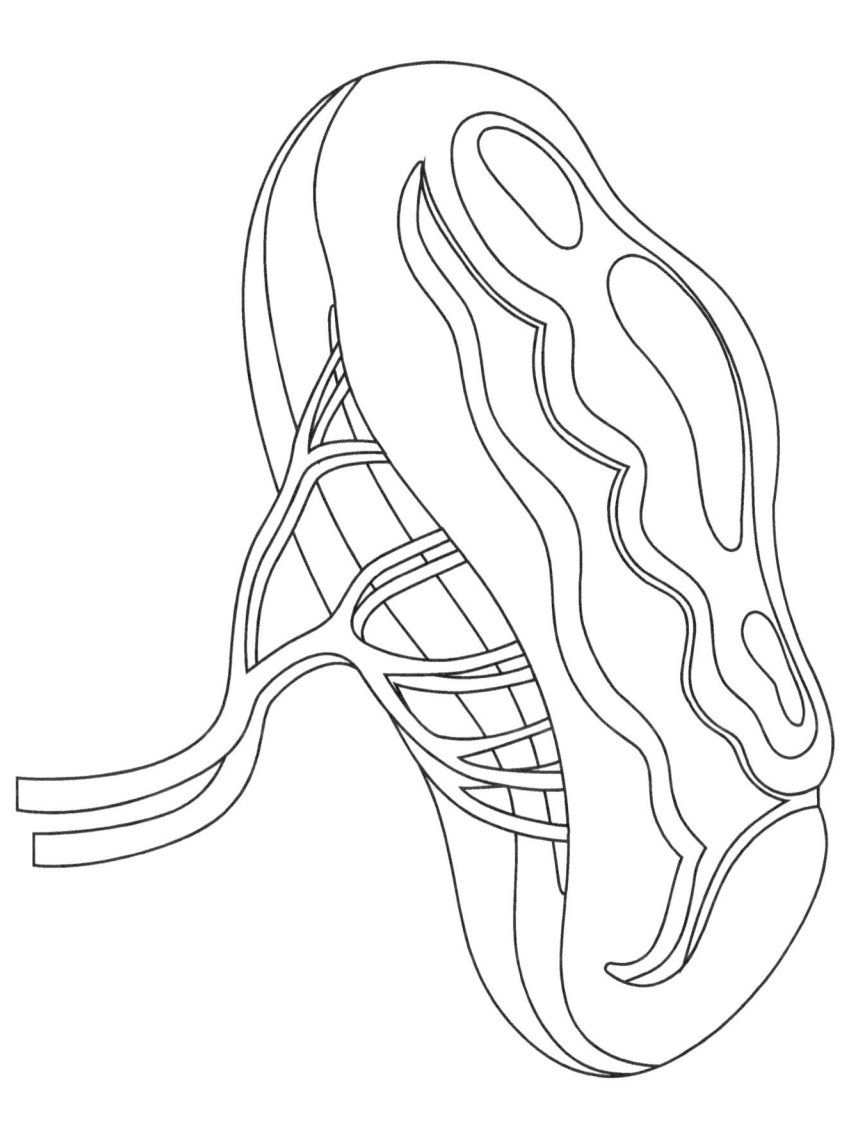

Spleen

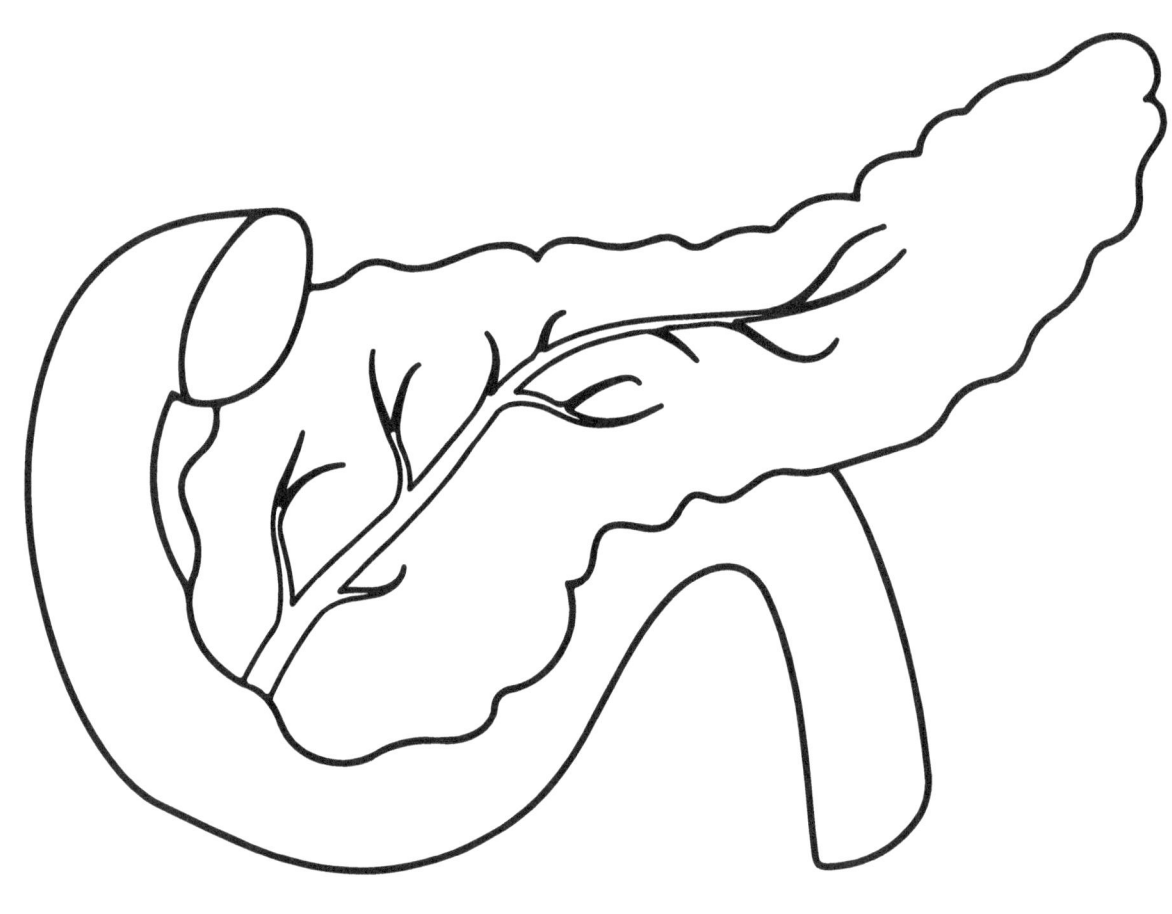

Pancreas

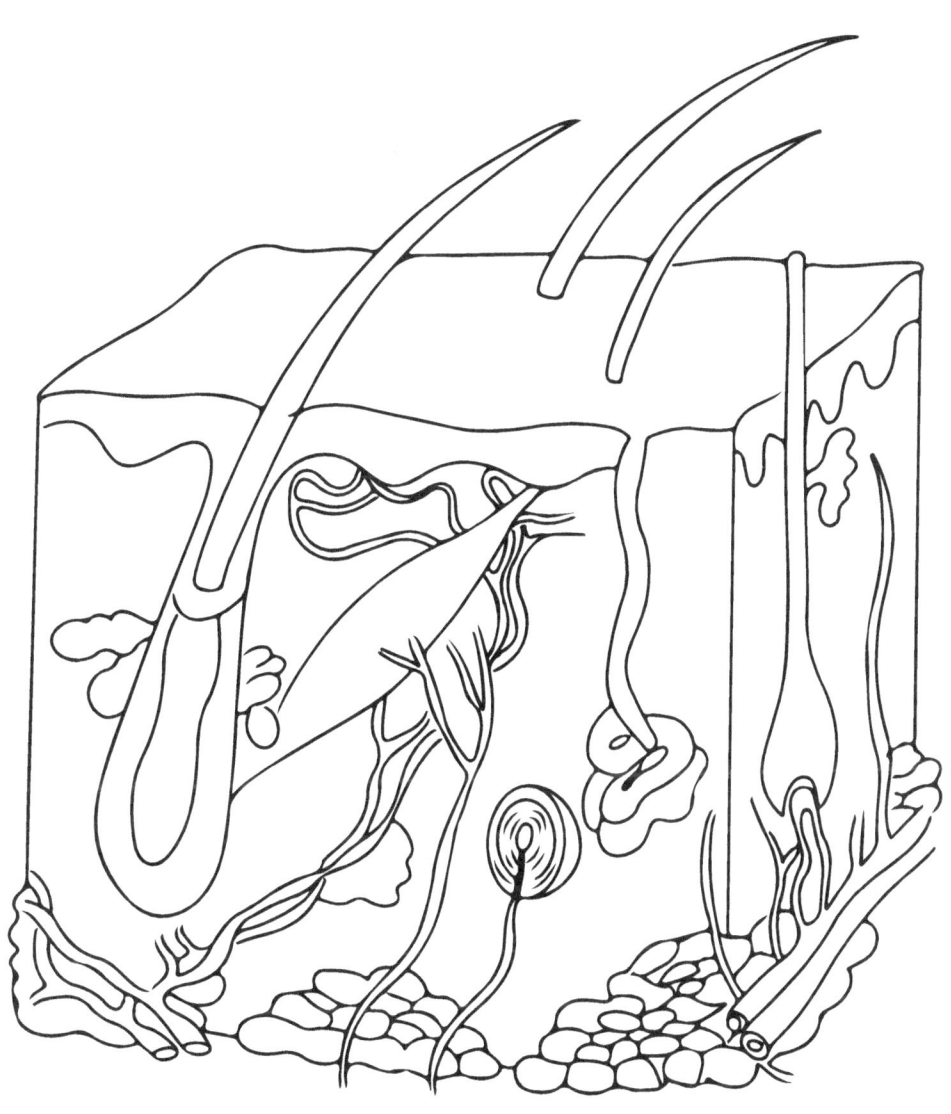

Skin

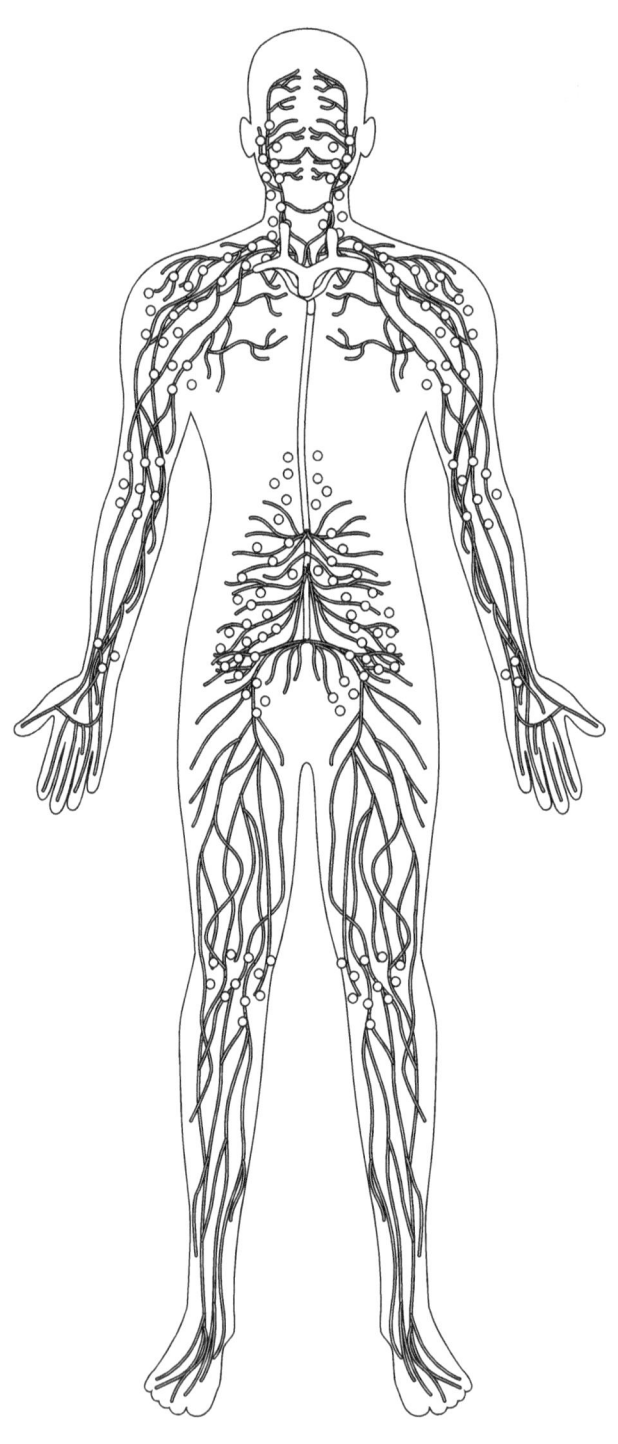

Lymphatic System

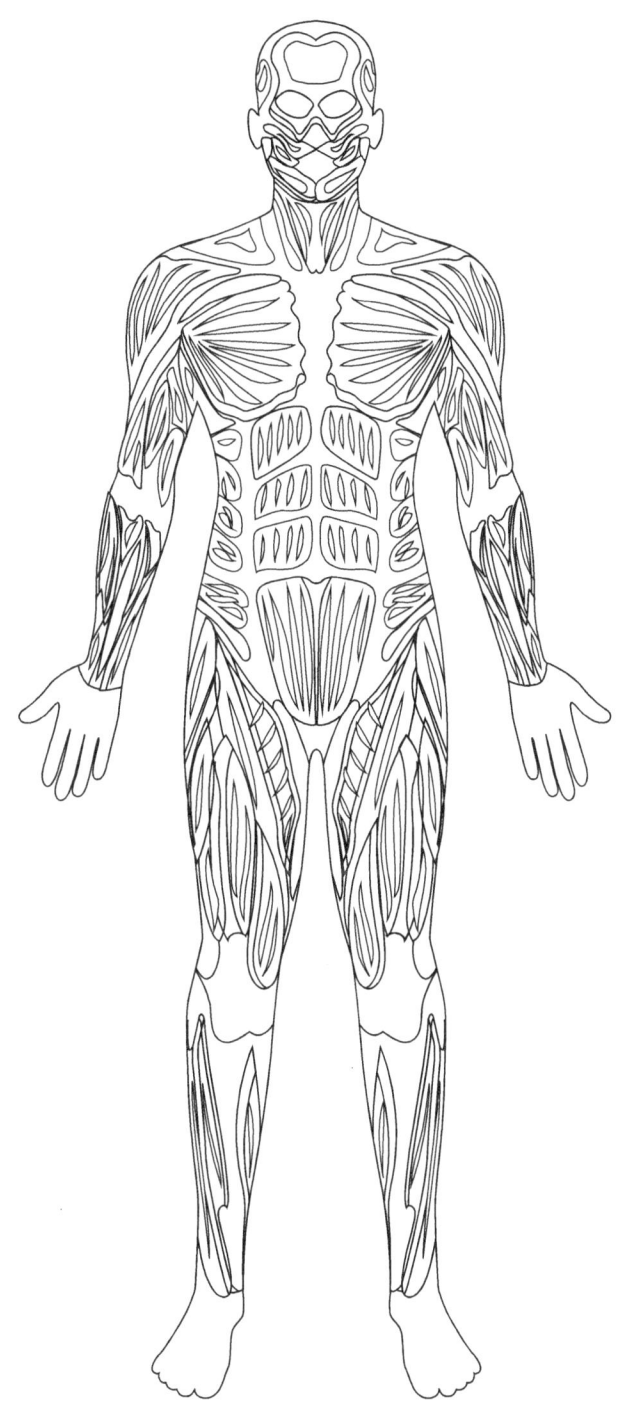

Muscle System

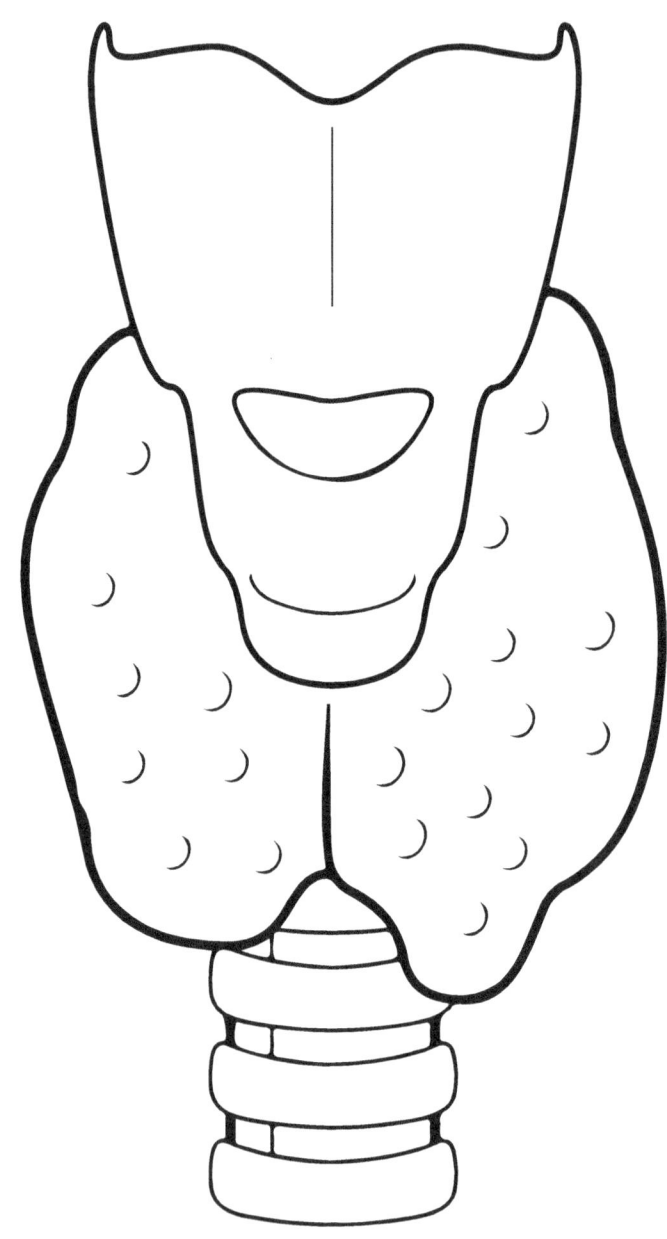

Thyroid